WHAT YOU MUST KNOW ABOUT
HASHIMOTO'S DISEASE

WHAT YOU MUST KNOW ABOUT
HASHIMOTO'S DISEASE

RESTORING THYROID HEALTH THROUGH TRADITIONAL AND COMPLEMENTARY MEDICINE

BRITTANY HENDERSON, MD, ECNU
ALLISON FUTTERMAN

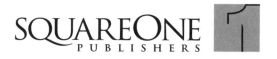

SQUAREONE
PUBLISHERS

COVER DESIGNER: Jeannie Tudor
IN-HOUSE EDITOR: Ally Cirruzzo
TYPESETTER: Gary A. Rosenberg

Square One Publishers
115 Herricks Road
Garden City Park, NY 11040
(516) 535-2010 • (877) 900-BOOK
www.squareonepublishers.com

This book is written in accordance to HIPAA privacy laws. All patient stories have been completely de-identified, names changed, and HIPAA rights protected. Allison Futterman has formally waived her HIPAA rights with regard to presenting her own medical information. All information is revealed to the audience in her own words throughout the book. The information and advice contained in this book are based upon the research and the personal and professional experiences of the authors. They are not intended as a substitute for consulting with a healthcare professional.

The publisher and author are not responsible for any adverse effects or consequences resulting from the use of any of the suggestions, preparations, or procedures discussed in this book. All matters pertaining to your physical health should be supervised by a healthcare professional. It is a sign of wisdom, not cowardice, to seek a second or third opinion.

Library of Congress Cataloging-in-Publication Data
Names: Henderson, Brittany Bohinc, author. | Futterman, Allison, author.
Title: What you must know about Hashimoto's disease / Brittany Bohinc
  Henderson, MD, ECNU, Allison Futterman.
Description: Garden City Park, NY : Square One Publishers, [2019] | Includes
  bibliographical references and index.
Identifiers: LCCN 2018040620 (print) | LCCN 2018050061 (ebook) | ISBN
  9780757054754 | ISBN 9780757004759 | ISBN 9780757004759¬q(paperback)
Subjects: LCSH: Hypothyroidism. | Autoimmune thyroiditis.
Classification: LCC RC657 (ebook) | LCC RC657 .H44 2019 (print) | DDC
  616.4/44—dc23
LC record available at https://lccn.loc.gov/2018040620

Printed in the United States of America

10   9   8   7   6   5   4   3   2   1

Contents

Acknowledgments

From Brittany Henderson, MD, ECNU

To the most important person in my life and my greatest gift from God— my husband, Jeff. Thank you for believing in me when I didn't even believe in myself. Thank you for listening to more thyroid facts than you would ever want to know and for always dreaming big with me. Your hugs and kisses were the fuel for my writing. You really are the wind beneath my wings. I love you!

To my family and friends, who have supported me throughout my life and my career. Mom, thank you for always answering my phone calls and for being my biggest prayer warrior. Dad, thank you for always keeping my email inbox full with the latest medical news articles. Ashley, Megan, Josh, Brooke, Beatrice, Ellis, Ken, Beverly, Lyn, Kathy, Uncle Dave, Gene, Jennifer, Ava, Logan, Riley and the rest of the family—I love you all! Thank you for allowing me to practice my thyroid exam on everyone year after year while sitting around the Thanksgiving dinner table. Kathryn, thank you for being my moral compass and best friend. Carly, Heather, Sarah, Irene, Jessica, Hannah, and Jennifer, thank you for keeping me laughing and for doing life with me. Grandpa and Grandma Bohinc, Grandma and Grandpa Woidtke, Aunt Carol, and Eddie Casino—I can't wait to see you again one day and celebrate!

To Allison, my co-author, patient, and friend. Thank you for being my partner in bringing much needed information on autoimmune thyroid disease to those who need it most. From finishing each other's sentences to working tirelessly towards our common goal of helping others, you have been the best co-author and writing partner I could have imagined working with.

To the entire team at Square One Publishers, thank you for believing in the book and for bringing it to fruition. Your work in healthcare publishing is really changing people's lives.

To all of my teachers, mentors, and supporters throughout medical school, residency, fellowship, and beyond, thank you for your wisdom and the time you took to teach me.

To my patients—past, present, and future. You have been and continue to be my inspiration and the greatest calling in my life. Your stories and lives have touched me more than you will ever know.

Above all, I would like to give thanks to Almighty God, who has blessed me with the opportunity to become a doctor and the privilege to see patients through His eyes. He knew what my life's calling would be before I ever considered it. Any and all glory belongs to Him.

From Allison Futterman

Sincere thanks and appreciation to my parents, who each in their own way, have helped me through many years of challenging health/medical situations. My father, who continually encouraged me along the experience of working on this book, as well as all of my writing. My mother, for too many reasons to list, but they are known. But most of all, for leading a life of compassion and kindness, to which I aspire. I love you both.

Michele S., for never giving up on me, even after all these years. And for insisting, "Yes, I do want to know what's going on!" If there are two lifetime friends more different yet so alike in the ways that matter, I'd like to know who they are.

Cathy A., for her wisdom and wit, and for conversations that always leave me thinking. Most importantly, for inspiring me by the way she lives her faith—with her actions and by example.

Mai-Lis B., for being a kind-hearted and supportive friend. A rare person who is genuinely happy for the triumphs and success of others.

Dr. Susan Levine, for listening when others didn't, and for sending me for that initial thyroid ultrasound!

Of course, Brittany Henderson, my doctor, co-author, and friend—someone whose medical knowledge and skill are matched only by her innate goodness as a human being. We were perfectly suited to work together on this collaboration, like-minded at every step.

Last, but certainly not least, Rudy Shur, Ally Cirruzzo, and everyone at Square One Publishers. Rudy, I'm grateful for your belief in us and this book, and for our shared goal of helping people.

Preface

I didn't know I would become a thyroid doctor until my second year of medical residency. It was one morning after a long shift of overnight call. I was about to rush home to catch a few hours of desperately needed sleep, when I received an invitation to work that afternoon with a local endocrinologist who had a strong interest in thyroid disease.

Something innate in me led me to proceed toward the endocrinologist's office. Once at the office, the attending doctor and I entered a dimly lit procedure room. A young woman sat cross-legged on the table, looking at us with tears in her eyes.

"Thank you. You changed my life," she said to the attending doctor.

He did? But how?

I would later learn that she had been struggling for years with symptoms of the most common thyroid disease: Hashimoto's. I would learn that many people, millions in fact, were struggling with the very same disease. Millions more suffered from other thyroid disorders and thyroid cancer. That day, seeing the effect on that patient's life, I knew what my calling was.

I love being a thyroid doctor. It's not just my job or my career; it's my passion. I have personally witnessed people get better, *many* people. I've seen the initial looks of despair and desperation; I've listened through the tears; I've given countless hugs and words of encouragement. And I've also witnessed many of those same patients reclaim their lives, enjoy renewed work success and satisfaction, and regain their sense of joy. By combining my clinical knowledge with caring guidance, I have helped numerous patients overcome their life-altering thyroid-related illness. And I want to help you, too.

I am an endocrinologist and medical doctor by training. I am *not* the stereotypical uncaring thyroid doctor you have read about in the online blogs and self-help books. I'm not close-minded about the treatment of thyroid disease, and I believe there are multiple effective strategies for treatment.

Strategies for Hashimoto's treatment and management need to be individualized and patient-specific. Too often, lab numbers, *not* individual patients, are treated. There are too many patients who don't have access to credible, up-to-date, scientific evidence that either supports or negates thyroid-specific diets, vitamins, supplements, and medical treatments. This critical information, which I provide to my patients on a daily basis, I would like to provide to you.

For the past ten years, I have been working alongside patients to help them achieve their best thyroid health. Over those years, I have seen many patients in second, third, or fourth consultations for uncontrolled hypothyroidism, Hashimoto's disease, Grave's disease, thyroid nodules, and thyroid cancer. A recent study done by the American Thyroid Association (ATA) found that over 45 percent of people changed thyroid doctors at least once, with 12 percent changing physicians up to ten times because they felt they were not receiving the care they needed.

As a medical doctor, I find this completely unacceptable. I understand the desperation in seeking out someone, anyone, who will listen and attempt to treat such a life-altering disease. Many patients come to me confused about what's wrong with them or, once they have a diagnosis about what they should be eating and how they should be treated. With all the information out there, it can get overwhelming and confusing. With this book, we will lay out a way forward for you. There is a way through, and although it isn't easy or simple, it is possible. You can feel better than you do now, and this book will help you get there.

Brittany Henderson, MD, ECNU,
Endocrinologist and Thyroid Specialist

I was used to feeling sick. For years, I'd dealt with a multitude of chronic health issues, which took an enormous toll on my body and spirit. I spent years seeking answers and help. My medical conditions took a long time to diagnose, and had me going from doctor to doctor in search of assistance. What I found, more often than not, was indifference and doubt. Along the way, I was ignored, insulted, and dismissed by more doctors than I can count. I was told I might have multiple sclerosis, lupus, or cancer. Other times, doctors implied that I was crazy, depressed, or just a complainer.

What I was and what I still am is a person dealing with chronic health issues. The impact on my life has been transformative. It's been frustrating and exhausting. The worst part of dealing with chronic illness is the uncertainty and unpredictability of daily life, not knowing from day to day, or even hour to hour how I would feel. There has not been one aspect of my life left unaffected by my health struggles, either professionally or personally. Like you, I know what it's like to deal with the exasperating search for medical help while struggling with illness.

At times I've felt discouraged and struggled for hope. Autoimmune illness ebbs and flows, characterized by flare-ups and more dormant periods. And flare-ups of one problem usually lead to a ripple effect. Since this has been my experience for years, it wasn't totally unfamiliar to me when I discovered I had a new illness to contend with: Hashimoto's disease.

Getting to that diagnosis took time and perseverance. I soon realized that not all endocrinologists are thyroid experts. I searched for someone who focused on thyroid issues, and that's when I found Dr. Henderson. She was the one to diagnose me with Hashimoto's. And while it was clear to me at our very first meeting that she had an enormous scope of knowledge, it was also clear that this was a complex condition that was not easy to understand.

As I did with every other medical issue, I approached Hashimoto's as a seeker of information. Frustratingly, the multifaceted elements of this complicated illness proved too much for me to wrap my brain around. In my quest to better digest all the related components of thyroid disease, I spent countless hours online and read several books. I emailed Dr. Henderson with questions and follow-ups. She patiently and compassionately answered me, but I knew that I needed a more comprehensive understanding.

I realized that if I had questions, concerns, and frustrations, endless other Hashimoto's patients must have similar experiences. I needed help, they needed help. . . *we* needed help! So, as a real-life physician and patient team, Dr. Henderson and I decided to compile the most important, up-to-date information necessary for Hashimoto's patients along all parts of their thyroid journeys.

This book was written with *you* in mind. Please know that we understand and want to help. We don't profess to have magic bullets or miracle cures, because despite what you might have heard, no such thing exists. But we have much to share with you that will hopefully make a positive difference in your life. When you're done reading this, you'll be armed with accurate information, sound advice, and actionable recommendations.

Working on this book, as is the case with any of my writing, has been difficult at times. It's a challenge to use your brain and body when you have chronic medical issues. There were times I had to write from bed. I say this not to be discouraging or negative in any way, but to let you know that even when we, as patients, must make adjustments because of our situations, it's worth it.

While having a lifelong autoimmune illness may cause us to feel less than our best, at times we can find solace in having fuller command of our condition. Knowledge is power, and gives us greater control over our bodies and our lives.

Allison Futterman,
Writer and Hashimoto's Patient

Introduction

As you may have already discovered, your health and well-being can be profoundly affected by a butterfly-shaped gland that is the size of a walnut and located at the front of the neck. "But how?" you may ask. The answer is through the production of *hormones*, or signals that travel from the thyroid to the rest of the body through the bloodstream. When working normally, the thyroid gland can keep the body functioning in peace and harmony—but when not functioning normally, the thyroid can have a devastating impact on your health.

Hashimoto's thyroiditis is the most common thyroid disorder, affecting 14 million people in the United States alone. Simply put, Hashimoto's is the underproduction of thyroid hormone, leading to the development of hypothyroidism. But the larger impact of this disease stems from it being an autoimmune disorder. In addition to causing hypothyroidism, Hashimoto's refers to a situation in which the immune system attacks the body, resulting in life-changing effects on your health.

Having Hashimoto's can and often does leave sufferers feeling incredibly sick, frustrated, and confused. It is a lifelong condition with symptoms that can fluctuate between intense, sudden "flare-ups" and remission, or stretches of time when the disease lies dormant. Understanding your condition will help you to achieve stable thyroid function, meaning fewer flare-ups and less active symptoms.

Maybe you or someone you care about has recently been diagnosed with Hashimoto's. Or perhaps you've been struggling with it for years, still unable to find the help and relief you need. Possibly you suspect you may have Hashimoto's based on symptoms and your own research, but haven't been officially diagnosed yet. Our hope is that this book will concisely and accurately give you the information you need to help understand and be proactive about this specific thyroid condition.

Hashimoto's can be debilitating, and sufferers need to know how to be an active participant in their own care. In order to understand your Hashimoto's symptoms (fatigue, muscle pain, weight gain, headaches, throat pain, difficulty concentrating, skin issues, and constipation, among others), you need to understand as much as possible about this complex disease. Once you do, you can then be an advocate for your own thyroid health—which will lead to better overall health. This book will give you the information you need to know about Hashimoto's, from diagnosis to treatment.

There is a multitude of books and websites out there about thyroid disease, offering different perspectives and advice. In fact, there's so much information out there that it may overwhelm you. In your quest for knowledge, you may find yourself reading contradictory information, creating confusion and frustration. Even worse, you may be embarking on your fact-finding mission while you feel depleted from struggling from the effects of thyroid disease. There are so many opposing viewpoints, nutritional supplements, and diets, that you could try all of them and still never exhaust the possibilities. That is where we come in. You need one central place for clarity and guidance, and this is it.

You and others like you are the reason we wrote this book. As a physician and real-life patient, we have joined together to provide a place for thyroid patients to turn for answers. The information you'll find here is grounded in both evidenced-based medicine (related to research findings) and clinical experience (based on treating thousands of patients). Our collaboration brings a uniquely valuable combination of a knowledgeable thyroid specialist and a patient who has been where you are.

There is no one-size-fits-all approach to thyroid disease, and that's because Hashimoto's is a multifaceted illness. The more you know, the greater impact you can have in reaching your personal best health. You need facts and a plan. That's what this book is here to do. We will guide you, step-by-step, along your journey to better thyroid health. We've written this book in a way that breaks down complicated medical issues into understandable concepts that will enable you to navigate the complex world of Hashimoto's.

The book is divided into three sections. Part 1 covers thyroid basics and is your introduction to why the thyroid is so important to your overall health. After reading Part 1, you will have a firm understanding of what autoimmune disease is and how it can affect the thyroid gland in particular.

We will also discuss thyroid nodules and thyroid cancer, two concurrent diseases that are more likely to occur in patients with Hashimoto's disease.

Part 2 is designed to explain the world of testing and diagnosis that lies ahead, which is of critical importance in Hashimoto's disease. We will discuss available thyroid blood tests and how they can be used to optimize your thyroid health, along with a variety of other important tests that can help to establish or confirm a diagnosis and yield pertinent information about your specific situation. We also walk you through the biopsy process and introduce you to the emerging area of molecular testing.

The last section of the book is all about Hashimoto's treatment and management. Here, we will provide extensive information about treatment, including thyroid hormone replacement options, integrative approaches, diets, supplements, and avoiding environmental exposures. We will provide useful tips on how to achieve optimal thyroid levels and suggest ways to avoid flare-ups. Finally, we will offer recommendations on credible resources where you can find a qualified thyroid specialist or supportive community of fellow patients who have already achieved success.

Our goal is to help you be an advocate and active participant in your own healthcare. While we can't say the process will be quick or easy, it will be worth it. Just know that many thyroid patients have been where you are today. Sick. Exhausted. Scared. Maybe even hopeless. But hang in there, because you aren't alone in this. There is help. And most importantly, there is hope.

PART 1

Getting to Know
Your Thyroid

1.

Thyroid Basics

Y ou had probably never thought about your thyroid until you started having thyroid problems, which makes sense, because the thyroid is usually not something given much consideration when your health is good. You typically become aware of your thyroid because there is some kind of issue that is either causing any number of symptoms, or because you receive an abnormal test result. If you are reading this book, this probably refers to you or someone important in your life.

In order to best understand thyroid disease, and specifically Hashimoto's, you first need to understand the fundamentals of the thyroid— what it is and what it does (or is supposed to do), the associated hormones and their functions, and how to interpret thyroid levels. In the following chapter, we will cover the thyroid basics. The information you learn here will lay important groundwork for the rest of the book and get you well on your way to understanding what you need to know about Hashimoto's disease.

GETTING TO KNOW YOUR THYROID

The thyroid is known as the "butterfly gland" because its shape resembles that of a butterfly. It is composed of a right lobe, left lobe, and a connecting middle portion called the isthmus. (See Figure 1.1 on page 8.) Up to 40 percent of people have a third, smaller pyramidal lobe extending up from the isthmus. Normal thyroid glands are difficult to feel, whereas abnormal glands can sometimes be felt within the neck.

You can feel your own thyroid gland by moving your fingertips down the middle portion of the front of your neck until you reach the chest bone. The thyroid gland is now located immediately below your fingertips. It is sometimes easier to feel if you swallow a sip of water, as the thyroid moves with swallowing.

There are various abnormalities that can be found by a medical professional when feeling the thyroid gland, such as enlargement, firmness, anterior neck pain, and nodules. In Hashimoto's disease, some patients note tenderness with palpation but can't feel anything structurally wrong with the gland, whereas others notice a sense of swelling. Hashimoto's disease is sometimes also referred to as Hashimoto's *thyroiditis*, which means inflammation of the thyroid.

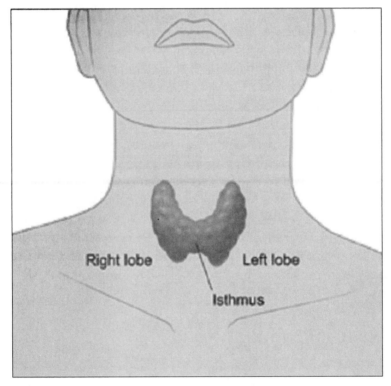

Figure 1.1. The Thyroid
Source: National Cancer Institute. Illustrator, Don Bliss.

Your primary care doctor, OB/GYN, and endocrinologist are all experts in detecting abnormalities in the thyroid gland. If you believe that your thyroid is enlarged, ask them for their opinion. Your lymph nodes, those small glands containing immune cells responsible for fighting off infection, can sometimes also be felt in the neck, usually by moving your fingertips from the ear down to the shoulder. Most often, lymph nodes are nothing to worry about, particularly if they feel tender. Lymph nodes are supposed to enlarge—it's their job! You may feel lymph node enlargement when you get sick, have allergies, or in the area under your jaw close to your mouth, where you are constantly exposed to bacteria. If you notice an enlarged lymph node, don't panic. Instead, ask your doctor for his or her opinion.

Check Your Neck

While you should not rely on self-diagnosis, you *should* have a high level of self-awareness as it relates to your body. Although we now have advanced methods, such as imaging tests and blood tests, the "hands-on" physical exam is still an important part of thyroid assessment.

Checking your own thyroid is simple and easy to do:

1. Get a mirror and a glass of water.

2. Focus on the area between your Adam's apple and the top of your breastbone.

3. Tilt your head back.

4. Take a sip of water.

5. As you swallow, look at your neck in the area above the breastbone and below the Adam's apple.

6. Look for lumps, protrusions, or fullness. Also take note of anything asymmetrical, where you only see the thyroid on one side and not the other.

7. If you feel lumps higher up under your jaw or chin or as you move your fingertips from your earlobe straight down to your collarbone, these are likely lymph nodes or swollen glands. Sometimes they can be tender. They are usually normal and can be reacting to allergies or recent infection. Always discuss your findings with your doctor.

8. If you have difficulty doing the test yourself, have someone help you by looking at your thyroid area while you tilt your head and drink the water.

If you suspect you have a thyroid problem, always seek professional attention.

BODY SYSTEMS AFFECTED BY THE THYROID

Your thyroid is a big deal. Even though it's small and located in your neck, the thyroid affects body parts from the top of your head to the tip of your toes. Through the production of hormones, the thyroid sends signals that travel throughout the body. Think of hormones as a set of instructions sent from the thyroid to all bodily cells telling them how to function normally. Because these hormones run throughout your bloodstream, they regulate functions in all other organ systems, including muscle, brain, liver, kidney, reproductive organs, bone, and almost every other body part you can think of. When those instructions are sent incorrectly, things go awry.

At the cellular level, thyroid hormones are important for many processes that regulate health. When functioning normally, the thyroid gland regulates and influences the following important bodily functions:

- Body temperature
- Bone health
- Brain function (wakefulness, energy, mood, and clear thinking)
- Cholesterol levels
- Gut motility and bowel function
- Heart health and blood pressure

- Kidney function and fluid retention
- Liver processing
- Metabolism and energy balance (your weight)
- Muscle function
- Reproductive health
- Sebaceous gland secretion (skin and hair health)

So, as you can see, the thyroid is one of the most important regulators of your health. When it malfunctions, many other symptoms can occur. In order to understand thyroid dysfunction, it is first important to understand how the thyroid works *normally* to produce and regulate thyroid hormones. When we get to Chapter 3, you'll see a list of the many problems associated with thyroid dysfunction.

THYROID REGULATION

In order to maintain normal thyroid levels, the body regulates and monitors thyroid hormones at multiple levels. These thyroid hormone "checkpoints," which act to keep the thyroid levels in balance, include the pituitary gland, various hormones and enzymes, and the thyroid gland itself. Thyroid health can become negatively affected when one or more of these "checkpoints" fail to function properly.

The Pituitary Gland

The thyroid gland is actually regulated by another gland called the *pituitary*, otherwise known as the "master gland." The pituitary gland, located within the brain, is the source of thyroid stimulating hormone, or TSH. TSH has one purpose: to tell the thyroid gland to make enough thyroid hormone. The pituitary gland produces more TSH when the thyroid gland is producing too little thyroid hormone, and less TSH when it's producing too much.

In the same way, the pituitary produces more TSH when thyroid replacement medicine—such as Armour or Synthroid, both of which will be discussed in Chapter 8—is too low, and less TSH when thyroid replacement medicine is too high. This process is known as "negative feedback" and, most of the time, it works perfectly.

Thyroid Cells

When the TSH signal from the pituitary reaches the thyroid gland, thyroid cells get to work making thyroid hormones. Think of the pituitary gland as the "boss," the thyroid gland as a "thyroid hormone-producing factory," and the thyroid cells as the "worker bees." When the worker bees get the green light from the boss, they react by first absorbing iodide (also called iodine, which is another chemical form of iodide) from the bloodstream. This is the first step in thyroid hormone production, and the first thyroid checkpoint.

Iodide

Wondering where the iodide comes from? Everyone has iodide, or the ion form of naturally occurring iodine, in his or her blood. The body's supply of iodide is derived from iodine-rich food sources like fish, seaweed, and iodized salt. Deep within the thyroid gland, iodide is processed and stored by different proteins and enzymes, two important parts of the thyroid factory's "machinery." More on the importance of iodide in Chapter 2.

T3 and T4

Imagine the thyroid "factory" operating along a conveyor belt. Two of the most important thyroid hormone-producing machines on the thyroid conveyor belt are thyroid peroxidase (TPO) and thyroglobulin (Tg). At the end of the conveyor belt, the two major forms of thyroid hormone, thyroxine (T4) and triiodothyronine (T3), are produced. This occurs after TPO takes iodide from the bloodstream, makes iodine, and attaches it to Tg to make T4 and T3. The Tg machine stores these pre-made thyroid hormones within the thyroid gland until it receives its orders from the pituitary boss, via TSH, to release T4 and T3 into the bloodstream. Once released, thyroid hormones travel throughout the body to regulate things like brain function, bowel function, and metabolism.

In the human thyroid gland, 80 percent of the thyroid hormone produced is T4, otherwise known as *inactive thyroid hormone*, and 20 percent is T3, referred to as *active thyroid hormone*. Said another way, the body normally produces T4 in T3 and a ratio of 4:1. This is an intentional function of the body, done in order to effectively regulate the amount of T3 your brain, liver, bone, muscle tissue, and other organs receive at one time. Ensuring that your body gets just the right amount of T4 and T3 is critical for maintaining your health. Too little T4 or T3, and you may feel muscle aches or notice hair loss; too much T4 or T3, and you may have heart palpitations, anxiety, and night sweats. That's why the body's thyroid hormone "checkpoints" are so important. They keep tight control over the amount of T4 and T3 your body sees at one time.

For example, when you were a fetus in your mother's womb, there were times when your body and placenta purposely decreased or increased all your available thyroid hormone to allow your organs and tissues to develop normally. Your body still works this way in adulthood. During times of illness or after a heart attack, for example, the body intentionally decreases thyroid hormone to allow time for your body to properly heal. Thyroid hormone production and regulation is one of the most important parts of optimal health.

Deiodinases (DIO)

As an adult, your body regulates your T4 and T3 levels with the help of enzymes called *deiodinases* (DIO), which function as another important thyroid checkpoint. There are different forms of DIO located throughout your muscle tissue, brain, liver, and kidney. These enzymes work together to convert the T4 produced by your thyroid gland into T3, active thyroid hormone. Proper function of your deiodinase enzymes is just as important as production of thyroid hormone from the thyroid gland itself. If your deiodinases are working properly, the cells throughout your body will see enough thyroid hormone in the form of T3.

If everything from your pituitary gland to your iodide supply to your DIO enzymes is working normally, production of thyroid hormone should run on autopilot. Metabolism, brain health, heart health, bone health, liver health, bowel function, fluid balance, and reproductive function should all operate normally.

UNDERSTANDING THYROID LEVELS

There is nothing more frustrating than receiving the results of your thyroid blood tests and having no earthly idea of what they mean. If you have Hashimoto's, it is important that you develop an understanding of the most pertinent thyroid indicators on your blood test results. You need to first understand the way these tests work—individually and together. We'll learn more about test results in Chapter 5.

What Is TSH and Why Is It So Important?

The pituitary gland produces thyroid-stimulating hormone in order to regulate the thyroid's production of T4 and T3. A TSH blood test is the most commonly performed thyroid test. Interestingly, the TSH test does not directly check your body's supply of thyroid hormone. Instead, it tests the pituitary gland's assessment of whether your thyroid factory is doing a good enough job producing thyroid hormone. Why not go straight to the source and check the actual thyroid levels, you may be asking yourself? Because TSH is a really good snapshot of what your body's been doing over the past month.

Think of TSH as the electric meter at your house. Read once a month, it can tell you how much total thyroid hormone you have produced in the month of February, for example, but it doesn't tell you how much you produced last Monday or will produce next Tuesday. Said differently, you may have months where you have exactly the same daily output of thyroid hormone, and months where you have one week of good thyroid output followed by several lousy weeks; in both cases, the TSH "read" at the end of the month may be the same. Thus, TSH is a "bird's-eye view" of your body's thyroid supply over time. It doesn't tell you everything, as you will come to find out, but it is an important piece of the thyroid puzzle.

The Rise and Fall of TSH

When the pituitary gland receives a signal that the thyroid gland isn't doing a good enough job, resulting in low thyroid hormone throughout the body, the pituitary produces more TSH. This increase in TSH levels is referred to as *hypo*thyroidism, meaning not enough thyroid hormone. Conversely, when the pituitary gland realizes that the thyroid gland is working overtime, producing too much thyroid hormone, it lowers TSH production. A low TSH level suggests *hyper*thyroidism, meaning too much thyroid hormone. The relationship between TSH and thyroid hormone is one of opposites, meaning that the higher the TSH number, the less thyroid hormone you are producing—and vice versa.

The Limits of TSH Testing

Overall, TSH is a good and reliable indicator of thyroid function. It is important to determine how your thyroid gland is doing overall, but TSH is not the only factor that is important in assessing thyroid health. In practice, we see plenty of patients with seemingly "normal" TSH levels who actually have a thyroid problem (more on this in Chapter 5). Conversely, we see patients with *truly* normal TSH levels who really do have normal thyroid hormone levels. Evaluating your TSH in a larger context, checking additional thyroid hormones, like T4 and T3, and assessing changes in your thyroid gland are all important in evaluating thyroid health.

T4 (Thyroxine) Levels

T4 is known as *inactive* thyroid hormone. Although inactive, it is crucial for your body to maintain a normal level of T4, because it drives production of T3, the active thyroid hormone, inside your cells. If your T4 level is too low, your liver, heart, and other tissues may not be "seeing" enough active thyroid hormone—even if your blood levels of T3 are normal!

T4 can be checked in one of two forms: total T4 or free T4. The total T4 includes both free T4, which is what your body can use right now, and stored T4, which is bound to proteins in your blood and saved for later use. We will discuss this in much greater detail in Chapter 5.

T4 Influences

Total T4 is influenced by many factors, and can be artificially increased or decreased by medications like birth control pills, hormone replacement therapies, or other medical issues. If your levels are high or low, it may not be anything to worry about. Be sure to ask your doctor. Free T4, on the other hand, measures the concentration of T4 currently available for use in the body. Levels of free T4 can also be influenced by medications, but to a lesser degree. In the normal human body, T4 is highly regulated and should not dramatically fluctuate from day to day or hour to hour.

In a healthy person, T4 is the most important thyroid hormone produced by the thyroid factory. As said, 80 percent of thyroid hormone production is T4, while only 20 percent is T3. Think of T4 as your body's bank account of thyroid hormone. When your heart, for example, needs more thyroid hormone to work properly, it will go to the bank and get out some T4 to make active thyroid hormone, T3. If your bank account is running low, tissue concentrations of thyroid hormone decrease. T3, on the other hand, is like the money in your wallet. It's easy to spend, but quickly wanes unless you have a bank account (T4) to back it up. We will dive further into the regulation and influences on T4 in Chapter 5.

T3 (Triiodothyronine) Levels

T3, the *active* form of thyroid hormone, is another important hormone level to have checked. If the T3 level is too low, patients may feel sluggish, complain of muscle aches, and experience continued hypothyroid symptoms. If T3 is too high, patients may experience hot flashes, heart palpitations, exercise intolerance, decreased energy (yes, decreased!), worsening anxiety, and hyperthyroid symptoms.

Like T4, T3 can be measured in two forms: total T3 and free T3. Total body T3 concentration not only relies on the health of the thyroid gland but, more importantly, on the proper function of deiodinase (DIO) enzymes throughout the body. In a healthy person, 80 percent of T3 is produced within the tissue itself by conversion of T4 to T3, *not* by the thyroid gland.

T3 Influences

While T3 testing does play an important role, current testing methods have limitations, which are important to understand. In addition to being influenced by birth control pills, hormone replacement therapy, and other disease states, similar to T4, T3 can be influenced by many other medications, foods, vitamin deficiencies, and acute illnesses. T3 regulation is extremely important for optimal thyroid health. We will discuss the regulation of T3 in much more detail in Chapter 5.

THYROID HORMONE PATTERNS

There are several thyroid patterns that can indicate a problem with the way your thyroid is functioning. People with abnormal thyroid patterns can be given a number of thyroid diagnoses, including hypothyroidism, subclinical hypothyroidism, hyperthyroidism, or subclinical hyperthyroidism. Many times, the distinction between subclinical and clinical thyroid disease can fall into a grey area. Because of this, many medical doctors disagree over whether to treat patients with levels in the subclinical range who have mild thyroid symptoms. For now we will review the standard definitions of these thyroid conditions, but we will dive deeper into this debate in Chapter 5.

Normal Thyroid Levels

Doctors like to call normal thyroid levels euthyroidism, which is a fancy way of saying, "Your thyroid labs are normal." In the euthyroid state, TSH, T4, and T3 will all be perfectly within normal ranges.

Hypothyroidism

In *hypothyroidism*, which is the main focus of this book, TSH rises because the pituitary gland doesn't sense enough thyroid hormone in the bloodstream. The hypothyroid patient's TSH will be high and T4 or T3 levels will be below normal reference ranges.

Hypothyroidism is a spectrum of disease, which means that there is a range of test values that are considered to be hypothyroid. When a patient is just starting to become hypothyroid, his or her TSH may be only slightly high or towards the top of the reference range, but technically still normal.

Additionally, T4 or T3 may be low-normal, but still within the normal reference range. This is sometimes referred to as "subclinical hypothyroidism," meaning below medical detection.

Subclinical Hypothyroidism

Think of subclinical hypothyroidism as hypothyroidism that is extremely mild. To be classified as "subclinical," you should not exhibit any symptoms of hypothyroidism. If you do have symptoms, you may still require treatment, even though some of your labs are in the normal range. Treatment of patients in this range is controversial in the medical literature and among medical practitioners. We will learn more about this issue in Chapter 5.

Hyperthyroidism

In *hyperthyroidism*, the pituitary gland stops making TSH because it detects too much thyroid hormone in the body. In hyperthyroid patients, TSH will be low and T4 and T3 high above the reference range. Again, hyperthyroidism is a spectrum of disease, with some patients having a TSH level that is undetectable (less than 0.1) and others having a TSH level just slightly below the normal range.

Subclinical Hyperthyroidism

Like subclinical hypothyroidism, subclinical hyperthyroidism is a slightly low TSH with normal T4 and T3. To be classified as subclinical, patients should have no hyperthyroid symptoms. Some medical guidelines recommend treating subclinical hyperthyroidism in patients over age sixty-five and in patients with certain medical problems such as osteoporosis and atrial fibrillation.

YOUR OWN THYROID PATTERN

In order to understand your thyroid pattern, it is important to know your full thyroid profile, which includes TSH, free T4, and free T3. Your thyroid laboratory pattern will provide clues about your thyroid function. As we will find out later, interpreting thyroid levels is not the only way to make a diagnosis of Hashimoto's disease. But it is a good place as any to start.

Each lab that does testing can have a slightly different range of what it considers normal, so always make sure you check the corresponding "normal reference range." You should be aware of where your numbers fall. Are they below the normal range? Above? Or do your results fall within the normal range? When we get to Chapter 5, we'll get into specifics about thyroid range goals—along with current controversies about what's considered normal. For now, what does your thyroid pattern say about you?

> *Thyroid Quick Tip:* It's best to interpret your TSH blood tests in context of your T4 and T3 levels. Is your body producing normal thyroid levels? Is it overproducing TSH in order to compensate for low amounts of thyroid hormone? Or is it under-producing TSH because your thyroid hormone levels are too high?

CONCLUSION

Although small in size, the thyroid gland plays a large role in your overall health. Your health and well-being is affected by thyroid hormone production. That is why it is necessary to understand the function of thyroid hormones, both individually and collectively.

Think of the thyroid gland as a factory that produces T4 and T3, under the ever-watchful eye of the pituitary gland. For effective thyroid function, you need four times as much T4 as T3, because that ratio allows the body to use active thyroid (T3), while giving it access to the reserve (T4) in the thyroid "bank." While T4 and T3 are different hormones, they work together, and when they malfunction, thyroid disease is the result. What happens when something goes wrong? We are about to find out.

2.

An Overview of Thyroid Disease

Thyroid disease and disorders have existed for thousands of years. Over time, there has been an evolution in the recognition, identification, and understanding of thyroid dysfunction. Here we will explore the history of thyroid problems and the underlying issue of Hashimoto's—autoimmunity. Having a basic understanding of thyroid disease—what it is, how it occurs, and what serious problems it can cause—is the next step in understanding Hashimoto's thyroiditis.

THYROID PROBLEMS THROUGH THE AGES

Thyroid disease has been in our history books for centuries. Historical Chinese texts have made references to goiter, or enlargement of the thyroid gland, as far back as 3600 BC. Chinese physicians, in fact, were the first to describe successful shrinkage of goiter using high iodide products, such as seaweed and burnt sea sponge. They were pioneers in prescribing dried animal thyroid (from sheep and pigs) as treatment to patients, though they didn't understand why these treatments worked.

The Role of Iodine

It wasn't until the 1800s that the importance of the mineral iodine in thyroid hormone production was understood. While hard at work making gunpowder in his laboratory, a scientist named Bernard Courtois incidentally noticed an unusual purple vapor arising from seaweed ash he had treated with sulfuric acid. This purple substance was later called iodine (named after the Greek word *ioeides*, meaning "violet-colored"), and

Da Vinci and the Thyroid

When you see or hear the name Leonardo Da Vinci, you probably think of masterpieces like the *Mona Lisa* or *The Last Supper*. But Da Vinci was also a pioneer when it came to artistic renderings of the human body. By dissecting cadavers, he was able to accurately depict human anatomy and the workings of the body. Over 500 years ago, in the year 1500, Da Vinci created the first drawing of the thyroid, recognizing it as an organ. Although he did not understand the function of the thyroid, he referred to it as a "gland" (interestingly, endocrine glands are also organs), which was visionary at the time.

Before Da Vinci's groundbreaking medical and artistic exploration of the thyroid (among many other areas of anatomy), nobody knew the gland existed. During the time of Hippocrates, ancient Greeks were aware of neck swelling, which later came to be known as goiter, but did not understand the anatomical structure from which it originated. They also mistakenly believed that contaminated water was the cause.

The all-important gland went unnamed until 1656, when British physician and anatomist Thomas Wharton coined it "thyroid." The name was based on the Greek word for "shield," based on the shape of the cartilage that protects the area around the thyroid.

formally introduced as a new element in 1813. By the 1890s, a German chemist named Eugen Baumann discovered a high concentration of iodine in the thyroid glands of both animals and man, concluding that iodine was essential for proper thyroid function.

Related to iodine is iodide, which is the same element in a different form, called an ion. The human body doesn't produce either iodine or iodide. We ingest foods with iodine, and a biochemical process then converts that iodine into its absorbable form: iodide. This is how we get a usable form of the necessary iodine needed for thyroid function.

Goiter

Soon thereafter, iodine deficiency was established as the basis of what's called "endemic goiter," or thyroid gland enlargement. It was found that, without enough dietary iodine, the thyroid gland would compensate by increasing in size to keep up with the body's demand for thyroid hormones. In cases where the gland ultimately couldn't grow large enough to produce sufficient amounts of thyroid hormones, the patient would develop hypothyroidism.

By the early 1900s, it was common to see goiters in people throughout the world, primarily due to deficiency of iodine in their diets. In fact, in early twentieth century American artwork and photography, adults, children, and even dogs were commonly depicted with enlarged thyroid glands.

Endemic goiter was especially prevalent in the "goiter belt," where up to 70 percent of people living in the Great Lakes, Appalachia, and Northwest regions of the United States had poor dietary exposure to iodide in saltwater seafood. Studies show that during the World War I draft, about 30 percent of Michigan registrants were documented as having enlarged thyroid glands, many of who were disqualified from enlisting due to goiter.

In 1917, an Ohio physician named David Marine conducted a study where he gave iodine to 2,100 schoolgirls. His findings surprised the medical community. Young girls given iodine had a significantly reduced frequency of goiters compared to children who did not receive iodine supplementation, reducing the incidence from one-fourth of kids affected to almost none. Dr. Marine's research established a correlation between the cause of goiter and its treatment.

On May 1, 1924, commercial salt companies began to add iodine to their manufactured salt products. Iodized salt became available on grocery shelves all over America, and widespread goiter dissipated. You might think that would have been the end of our thyroid dilemma, but it was not. So why do so many people still have thyroid problems?

AN EPIDEMIC OF AUTOIMMUNITY

While the widespread availability of iodine helped one problem, there was a larger problem looming menacingly on the horizon—that of modern civilization. As science advanced further, eradication of numerous serious diseases through immunization and improved hygiene took an even greater toll on the thyroid gland in the form of autoimmunity, or "reaction to self."

What do we mean by *autoimmunity*? Your immune system is composed of white blood cells called lymphocytes, which protect you from infection and illness from viruses, bacteria, mold, and parasites. You were born with the innate ability to fight off foreign invaders to keep you safe. As you grew, your body learned to fight off new foreign invaders and developed something called the *adaptive immune response*. If you get a sinus or ear infection, for example, your immune system takes action, and you notice a stuffy nose and ear pain. If you get a virus, like the flu, for example, you may develop a high fever. Once the bacterial or viral infection has been defeated, your immune system will relax and sink into the background, patrolling the corridors of your body as it silently waits for its next major offender.

In autoimmunity, the immune system gets confused and incorrectly recognizes your own cells as foreign invaders. In response, it sends in an army of soldiers in the form of specialized white blood cells to attack your own thyroid cells.

This doesn't just happen in the thyroid gland; in fact, there are many other autoimmune diseases directed at various parts of the body. For example, Crohn's disease is an autoimmune disease of the intestine, alopecia is an autoimmune disease of the hair follicle, and multiple sclerosis is an autoimmune disease of the nervous system.

The National Institutes of Health estimates that up to 24 million Americans have autoimmune diseases. The American Autoimmune Related Diseases Association estimates an even higher number—up to 50 million Americans. Guess which autoimmune disease is among the most common? Autoimmune thyroid disease! So why have our immune systems gone awry?

The Hygiene Theory

In March 1819, a physician named John Bostock used his own situation as a test case. He presented himself to the Medical and Chirurgical Society of London, describing "a periodical affection of the eyes and chest." His report was the first to describe immune dysfunction in the form of hay fever. He noted that, while common among the upper class, he had not heard of a single case of hay fever occurring among the poor. Even more fascinating was that farmers, who were routinely exposed to pollens and environmental allergens, had the least amount of cases. Further research around the world confirmed "the farming effect."

Children from full-time farming families had half the allergies of those who were exposed to farming intermittently, and one-fourth the allergies of children who had no farming exposure. Pigpens, horse stalls, and stables were brimming with bacteria and environmental exposures that were, in turn, helping to prime the immune systems of these children, allowing them to become more tolerant of the world around them, thereby reducing allergies. Even infants whose mothers were exposed to barns and stables routinely *in utero* were born with a significant reduction in environmental allergies and autoimmune disease.

So, how does this translate to the current rise in thyroid disorders?

The most commonly accepted hypothesis is that the eradication of certain environmental exposures prevented proper development of our immune system to the world around us. Instead of spending our days in stables and pigpens, we remain inside in the comfort of our own sterile environments. Eradication of viruses (smallpox, for example), bacteria (malaria, tuberculosis), and parasites (hookworm, ringworm) in modern society, as well as dust mites and tree pollens with integration of our air purifying systems, has left our immune systems improperly trained to fight off infection. Without a properly trained immune system, our soldiers are essentially fighting with blindfolds on. They can't accurately identify the enemy.

This theory (referred to as the "hygiene theory") is supported by several current studies examining allergies and autoimmunity. The explanations for this immune system vulnerability that are most widely agreed upon are: one, inadequate immune training early in life due to lack of breastfeeding or exposure to dirt and the outside environment in early childhood; two, living in sterile environments throughout life; and three, exposure to new viruses, artificial flavorings, environmental chemicals, and highly processed foods. In the latter situation, the already confused immune system is even further mistaken by incorrectly identifying these chemicals and artificial ingredients as "thyroid-like." Then, instead of attacking the real invader, the immune system attacks the thyroid gland itself.

AUTOIMMUNE THYROID DISEASE

As we mentioned previously, autoimmunity can result in many different diseases. In Crohn's disease, the immune system may identify the foreign invaders as "intestinal-like" and attack the gut. In alopecia, the immune system may fight off hair follicles, resulting in hair loss. The same goes for multiple sclerosis, where the immune system attacks the brain and nervous system.

The thyroid is an especially easy target of attack by the immune system, although we do not yet know why. What we *do* know is that with the eradication of iodine deficiency and modern medicine's move towards disease prevention and increased sterility, another thyroid-specific endemic was born—that of autoimmune thyroid disease, commonly referred to as AITD.

The Two Types of Autoimmune Thyroid Disease

There are two major classes of autoimmune thyroid disease (AITD): Hashimoto's thyroiditis and Graves' disease, both named after the doctors who first identified them.

Hashimoto's typically takes the form of hypothyroidism, while Graves' is associated with hyperthyroidism. While you may be most concerned with Hashimoto's-induced hypothyroidism, it's important to know about both forms of AITD, because there can be a major overlap between the two.

Think of AITD as a spectrum of disease (similar to the autism spectrum). There are some patients that have severe hypothyroidism, some that have severe hyperthyroidism, and some that toggle back and forth between the two. The resulting thyroid disease is largely dependent on what the immune system is doing at the moment. Therefore, it is best to think of AITD as an immune system problem, rather than a problem with the thyroid gland itself.

Thyroid Quick Tip: Autoimmune thyroid disease is a disease of the immune system, *not* the thyroid.

The Immune System

To better understand AITD, it is important that we examine the immune system a little more in depth. In AITD, the immune system incorrectly detects the thyroid gland as a foreign invader and launches an attack against it. There are two major classes of immune cells that we need to know about: T cells and B cells. T cells are similar to army foot soldiers. In thyroid disease, they march into the thyroid gland and go to hand-to-hand combat with the thyroid cells, preventing them from carrying out normal thyroid hormone production.

B cells, on the other hand, are like snipers. Working together with the T cells, B cells use bullets called "antibodies" to disrupt thyroid hormone

Dr. Hashimoto—
The Man Who Identified the Disease

Dr. Hakaru Hashimoto started practicing medicine in Japan in 1907. For several years, he studied thyroid tissue samples he extracted from surgical patients, and noticed new characteristics not previously discovered. He found that thyroid samples in four women with goiter (all over the age of forty) had thyroid tissue that was infiltrated by lymphocytes, a type of white blood cell involved in fighting infection. Lymphocytes represented a new type of thyroid disease, distinct from other types of inflammation of the thyroid—referred to in medical terms as *thyroiditis*. In 1912, his findings were published in a German medical journal, in an article entitled, "Notes of lymphomatous in the thyroid gland (struma lymphomatosa)." This impactful work, which was published when he was thirty-one, was his only paper on the thyroid.

Dr. Hashimoto went on to further his medical training in Germany, but when World War I started, he returned to Japan. There, he worked as a physician until his untimely death at the age of fifty-two, caused by typhoid contracted from a patient.

Because his thyroid research had been published in German, the news of his discovery remained largely unknown throughout Japan and the rest of the world. It didn't gain attention until the mid-1930s, when a surgeon from the Cleveland Clinic, Allen Graham, confirmed Hashimoto's theory. Eventually, Hashimoto's name became inextricably associated with the disease he discovered, although unfortunately, he never received the credit or recognition he deserved during his lifetime. Other researchers, building upon his discovery, found antibodies associated with Hashimoto's disease, which cemented its (previously unknown) autoimmune connection.

The saying, "Medicine is a benevolent art," is attributed to Dr. Hashimoto, and it is a sentiment he put into practice. Devoted to his patients, he was a doctor that went above and beyond in his medical care, often traveling far distances by rickshaw to see patients throughout the Japanese countryside. Now revered in Japan, Dr. Hashimoto's portrait is used as the logo for the Japanese Thyroid Association.

production at the thyroid factory. In Graves' disease, for example, the B cells shoot off bullets called *TSH receptor antibodies* (TRAbs) that mimic the pituitary gland's secretion of TSH, which then increases thyroid hormone production and causes hyperthyroidism. In Hashimoto's thyroiditis, the B cells shoot off two different kinds of antibodies, named for each of the "machines" heavily involved in thyroid hormone production that they are responsible for attacking: *thyroid peroxidase antibodies*, or TPOAb, and *thyroglobulin antibodies*, or TgAb.

In all types of AITD, the T and B cells launch an attack on the thyroid gland, causing persistent thyroid inflammation, scarring, and development of thyroid disease. Having extra antibodies (bullets flying) can contribute to disease outside of thyroid dysfunction as well. This is commonly found with Graves' eye disease, where TRAbs cause growth and inflammation to the muscles at the back of the eye, causing eyes to bulge. There is also a school of thought that Hashimoto's antibodies (TPOAbs and TgAbs) can worsen depression and muscle pain in fibromyalgia, although further studies are needed. AITD patients typically experience multiple life-changing symptoms due to the disruption of normal thyroid function. We will explore all of this in greater detail throughout the remainder of the book.

THYROID NODULES IN AITD

Because of the constant war waging within the thyroid gland, AITD patients are prone to developing thyroid nodules. These are growths that occur within the thyroid gland itself. Some nodules may be large enough that you or your doctor may feel them by physical exam, but most are found accidentally on scans done for other reasons. Because many nodules are unable to be felt, some physicians choose to screen their AITD patients for nodules with a thyroid ultrasound. This is one area where a thyroid specialist may differ from a general endocrinologist, since he or she should be well-versed in nodules, and therefore extremely familiar with troublesome findings that may need to be carefully followed or treated.

Nodules on your thyroid are extremely common in both AITD and in healthy people. In fact, we think that up to 65 percent of the United States population has them. Your chance of developing a thyroid nodule increases with age. A good general rule is the likelihood of having a thyroid nodule is about the same percentage as your age (for example, 30 percent of thirty-year olds, 40 percent of forty-year-olds, and so on). Luckily, over 95 percent of thyroid nodules are benign—that is, not cancerous. Nodules can run in families or develop spontaneously. If you have more than one nodule, your practitioner may refer to your thyroid as a "multinodular goiter," or enlarged thyroid as a result of multiple nodules. Most nodules can be safely monitored over time by having regular ultrasounds, but some need a fine needle aspiration biopsy. We will discuss thyroid ultrasound and biopsy in the assessment of nodules in much greater detail in Chapters 6 and 7.

Unfortunately, although the majority of nodules are benign, abnormal AITD glands are associated with an increased risk for cancerous nodules. Increased risk for cancer is believed to be due to constant inflammation within the gland and elevated TSH levels in Hashimoto's disease. Because TSH stands for "thyroid stimulating hormone," elevated TSH "stimulates" underlying cancerous nodules to grow.

THYROID CANCER IN AITD

Today, thyroid cancer is the fastest growing cancer in this country. It is currently the fourth most common cancer in women. The growing incidence of AITD is one contributing factor to the increasing incidence of thyroid cancer, although genetics and environmental exposures also play a part. By genetics, we mean you may have a higher likelihood of thyroid cancer if a family member has been diagnosed. Other reasons for increased chance of thyroid cancer include exposure to radiation therapy—not just X-ray—or growing up in an area with nuclear fallout or radioactive materials. Emerging studies suggest a possible connection between lifelong exposure to flame retardant chemicals in your home and on your electronic equipment to the development of thyroid cancer.

Thankfully, the vast majority of people diagnosed with thyroid cancer have an excellent prognosis, with a 99 to 100 percent likelihood of long-term survival. For reasons yet unknown, men and older patients do much worse than women and younger patients who are less than forty-five years of age.

There are several types of thyroid cancer: papillary, follicular, medullary, and anaplastic. Of these, papillary thyroid cancer is the most common, with over 80 percent of cases falling into this category. Additionally, papillary thyroid cancers have different subtype classifications with technical-sounding names. It is important to know the cancer subtype to help predict tumor behavior. The other types of thyroid cancer are much more rare, and beyond the scope of this book. However, more information regarding these cancers is listed in the Resources section. (See page 239.)

If you or a loved one has a thyroid nodule, it is important that it be evaluated by a doctor with thyroid expertise. Many endocrinologists who specialize in thyroid disease or cancer can now perform ultrasounds and biopsies in their offices. This book will give you the tools you need to properly identify these physicians and seek the best thyroid care available.

CONCLUSION

As we have learned, thyroid problems have plagued people throughout the ages, long before thyroid disease was identified. As research and science has evolved, we now know that the thyroid gland is especially susceptible to disease.

What was once a dietary problem of iodide deficiency has now become a rampant problem of autoimmunity. Along with autoimmunity, we have identified a rising incidence of thyroid nodules and cancers. With the high prevalence of thyroid-related disease, it is important to be aware of potential thyroid problems, so you can address them early if you find yourself experiencing signs or symptoms. While we have touched on the basics of thyroid autoimmunity, the next chapter will explore the most common type of AITD: Hashimoto's thyroiditis.

3.

Hashimoto's Thyroiditis

Now that you know the basics about your thyroid and have a general understanding about thyroid disease, we'll move on to the issue directly affecting you or someone you care about: Hashimoto's thyroiditis. Because Hashimoto's is an autoimmune disease, it affects many aspects of health. There are seemingly endless symptoms Hashimoto's can bring about, which might be dismissed by the patient and even some doctors. As you read, you will learn that there are certain triggers and causes of Hashimoto's, and some people are more likely to develop it than others. Understanding the numerous facets of Hashimoto's is an integral part of reclaiming your thyroid health.

A HASHIMOTO'S STORY

Let's start with the story of Mrs. Jones, an energetic, fifty-two-year old "go-getter" who avoided doctors as much as she could. Throughout her entire adult life, she maintained good health, took vitamins, and followed a well-balanced diet. She exercised regularly and kept herself at a healthy weight. Then, one day, she woke up with tenderness at the front of her neck. She could not remember injuring the area, but had recently returned from an overseas trip. She thought she might have pulled a neck muscle.

In the days that followed, she noticed other symptoms: difficulty swallowing, brain fog, and overwhelming fatigue. Once someone who routinely got up with her alarm at 6:00 a.m., she now struggled to get out of bed by 10:00 a.m. She also noticed a swelling at the base of her neck, the site of her pain.

In an effort to find out what was happening to her, she did what we all do—she "Googled" her symptoms. She tried to switch her vitamins and alter her diet, but nothing was working, and she was getting worse. To her dismay, she was gaining weight, losing her hair, and noticed unflattering changes to her skin and nails.

She knew there was something very wrong, but perhaps out of fear, still hesitated to call her physician. However, with the increase of noticeable symptoms, she finally called and made an appointment to see her doctor.

Two days later, she received a phone call: "You have an underactive thyroid and positive testing for Hashimoto's." With all of her reading on the Internet, she had suspected it to be cancer, so she was relieved to find out it wasn't. She finally had a diagnosis, and she thought she'd just take a pill and all would be right with the world again. Easy—right?

Wrong. As many come to find out, a Hashimoto's diagnosis is not always as easy as it would seem. Yes, taking thyroid hormone replacement medicine helps, but Hashimoto's symptoms have a way of creeping up on you when you least expect them. Working diligently with your thyroid doctor as a partner in disease management, recognizing your symptoms, and understanding disease triggers is of utmost importance.

If you or a loved one has been diagnosed with Hashimoto's disease, you need to first understand what symptoms you are looking for.

UNDERSTANDING HASHIMOTO'S SYMPTOMS

Not everyone with Hashimoto's disease experiences the same list of symptoms. Hashimoto's can affect patients differently due to a variety of factors, including genetics (how you, as an individual, respond to illness), underlying vitamin or nutrient deficiencies, and your individual "root cause" of Hashimoto's (something we will discuss later in the chapter).

Symptoms are first broken down into three categories:

1. Hypothyroid symptoms, meaning the thyroid gland is underperforming.

2. Hyperthyroid symptoms, meaning the thyroid gland is overperforming.

3. Both hypothyroid and hyperthyroid symptoms.

For the specific symptoms of each, see Table 3.1. on page 32.

Remember, in the previous chapter, we mentioned that autoimmune thyroid disease is a spectrum, with people experiencing a wide array of associated symptoms. Also, the category of symptoms that you have now may not be the category of symptoms you experienced two years ago, and may be different from the symptoms you will experience in the upcoming years. That is to say, Hashimoto's symptoms can evolve or change with time.

Thyroid Quick Tip: With Hashimoto's disease, you can experience both hyperthyroid and hypothyroid symptoms, and your symptoms can change over time.

Identifying Your Symptoms

To make it as easy as possible, we have listed symptoms categorically as hypothyroid or hyperthyroid symptoms. Identifying your most frequent symptoms (and whether you are predominantly hypothyroid, hyperthyroid, or both) is important in understanding your unique Hashimoto's pattern.

Look for symptoms that are different. When identifying symptoms, it is important to only check off symptoms that are *different* than what you experienced when your body was healthy. For example, if you have been constipated your whole life and your bowel movements haven't changed, attributing the symptoms of constipation to a thyroid problem may be inaccurate. On the other hand, if you have had longstanding constipation with bowel movements twice weekly, but over the last several months are experiencing bowel movements twice monthly, then that is a significant change that may be attributed to your underlying thyroid condition.

Be selective in identifying your symptoms. All of us experience a majority of these symptoms at various times in our lives. We are looking for unusual symptoms that are new and persistent. When identifying your thyroid-specific symptoms, ask yourself, "What minor ailments do I experience consistently on a daily or weekly basis?" and "Which symptoms are different than the ones I had when I was healthy?"

Now that you've identified your symptoms, you should notice a pattern—let's call it your *Hashimoto's signature.* You may have symptoms only in the hypothyroid column or hypothyroid column, possibly with a few in the middle column, or you may have symptoms checked off in every column! This collection of symptoms may be very different from the symptoms your friend or family member with Hashimoto's experiences. This raises the question: Why do patients experience Hashimoto's disease so differently?

TABLE 3.1. LIST OF HASHIMOTO'S SYMPTOMS		
HYPOTHYROID SYMPTOMS	**CAN BE SEEN IN BOTH**	**HYPERTHYROID SYMPTOMS**
❏ Brain fog	❏ Easy bruising	❏ Anxiety and panic attacks
❏ Cold intolerance	❏ Extreme fatigue	❏ Diarrhea
❏ Constipation	❏ Difficulty swallowing	❏ Dizziness and vertigo
❏ Depression	❏ Hair loss	❏ Emotional rollercoaster
❏ Dry hair	❏ Throat pain or fullness	❏ Exercise intolerance
❏ Dry skin		❏ Extreme hunger
❏ Fluid retention		❏ Eye changes (pain, pressure, dryness, change in appearance)
❏ Headaches and migraines		
❏ Heavy or irregular periods		❏ Fever (usually low grade)
❏ Infertility		❏ Heart racing or skipping a beat
❏ Low body temperature		
❏ Muscle aches and cramping		❏ Heat intolerance
❏ Nail changes (broken, peeling)		❏ Insomnia
		❏ Night sweats (*unrelated to menopausal hot flashes*)
❏ Poor concentration		
❏ Puffy face		❏ Racing thoughts
❏ Recurrent miscarriage		❏ Shortness of breath (with exercise)
❏ Thinning eyebrows (the outside portion, in particular)		
		❏ Tremor (shaking)
❏ Weight gain		❏ Weight loss or inability to gain weight

HASHIMOTO'S DISEASE:
A DISEASE OF MANY ROOT CAUSES

Hashimoto's disease is a disease of autoimmunity. It has many root causes. The immune system can be triggered by a variety of different causes, such as:

- allergens
- drugs
- stress
- toxins
- processed foods
- infections

All of these triggers can cause differing immune reactions. Additionally, people who get AITD have different genetic make-ups that predispose them to various forms of Hashimoto's, all with different symptoms.

Allison's Experience: Listen to Your Body

Feeling sick was nothing new to me. Muscle and joint pain, migraine headaches, sore throats, chills, fatigue, and brain fog—for years, I've had them all. When I first got sick many years ago, I went from doctor to doctor in my search for help, before finally being diagnosed with chronic fatigue syndrome (CFS) and fibromyalgia.

Years later, when I felt an increase in all my usual symptoms along with throat pain and pressure in my neck, I *listened*. Again, it took perseverance on my part. I went to different doctors until I finally got an ultrasound of my thyroid, which led to the discovery of nodules. That led me on my quest to find an endocrinologist who specialized in thyroid disorders. There weren't any in my city or neighboring cities. But I was committed to finding the right doctor, which turned out to be Dr. Henderson. She went over my medical history; did an exam, ultrasound, and biopsy; and ordered blood tests and a thyroid uptake scan—ultimately leading to her diagnosis of Hashimoto's.

While it was upsetting to discover I had another illness to contend with, I was relieved to have answers. You, too, need to listen to your body. If a doctor doesn't take your concerns seriously, keep looking. If a doctor makes you feel uncomfortable, be willing to go elsewhere. Having a doctor who truly is your partner in health and listens to your perceptions and feedback is one of the greatest assets you will ever have in your journey to wellness.

Baby, You Were Born This Way

If you have Hashimoto's disease, odds are that you have at least one family member who also has the disease. Because it is eight times as common in women than in men, it is much more likely that your mother or grandmother had Hashimoto's, although fathers can pass it down, too. In fact, up to half of your siblings may have positive AITD antibodies (even if their TSH is normal!), and about one-third likely already have the disease.

Children and grandchildren can also get Hashimoto's. Thyroid disease in children isn't always identified in a timely manner. Many times, it reveals itself as poor school performance, depression, excessive sleeping and fatigue, or weight gain. For families that have multiple members affected by Hashimoto's disease, some thyroid doctors recommend that school-aged children ten and older be screened for an abnormal TSH level and thyroid peroxidase antibodies (TPOAbs).

It All Starts With Your Genes

What is a gene, anyway? A gene is the basic unit of what makes you uniquely *you*. Your genes were inherited, half from your mother and half from your father. Genes are made up of tiny, spiral-shaped molecules called DNA. Think of DNA as a set of instructions that tell your body how to function throughout your life. The DNA given to you from your mother and father may have specific genes that increase your risk of getting Hashimoto's disease or other autoimmune diseases later in life.

Ethnic Differences in AITD

Because genes play a significant part in autoimmune thyroid disease, it stands to reason that there are ethnic differences in those who develop various autoimmune diseases. Graves' disease, for example, is much more common in Black and Asian/Pacific Islander people than it is in Caucasians. Conversely, Hashimoto's disease is significantly more common in Caucasians.

THE DEVELOPMENT OF HASHIMOTO'S

The development of Hashimoto's can be thought of as a three-step process. This involves specific genes, environmental triggers, and a sustained autoimmune response. They build on each other, ultimately resulting in Hashimoto's. If a person does not experience all three, the process is interrupted along the way, and there will not be a culmination in Hashimoto's. When you understand the three-step process, you will grasp how Hashimoto's develops.

STEP ONE: Hashimoto's-Specific Genes

So which genes exactly play the biggest role in AITD? The origin of Hashimoto's lies with Hashimoto's-prone gene sets. The first gene set is thyroid-specific; the second, and likely more important, involves genes that control the immune system.

The immune genes have two important jobs in the body: one, keeping peace and identifying your thyroid cells as part of you; and two, deciding when to go to war by sending fighter T cells (or combat foot soldiers) into the thyroid gland.

When the genes you inherited from your mom and dad start misbehaving and giving off the wrong signals, they can contribute to development of AITD. We don't routinely check people for these specific gene sets because we don't know how to treat them, but it is significant to know that Hashimoto's is a disease that begins with your genes. These Hashimoto's-prone gene sets can also increase your risk for developing other autoimmune diseases. (We will cover this in more detail in Chapter 4.)

STEP TWO: Environmental Triggers in Autoimmune Thyroid Disease

Not everybody with a Hashimoto's-prone gene set gets AITD. In fact, we see patients all the time that can't identify a single relative with thyroid disease, yet they have Hashimoto's themselves. The most likely thing is that one or more of their parents have the susceptibility gene(s) but never were exposed to step two in development of AITD: exposure to an *environmental trigger*. In fact, exposure to an environmental trigger may be much more important than your genetic susceptibility in developing AITD.

Along the way, you or your loved one was exposed to a virus, bacteria, or environmental/food allergen or toxin that triggered an inflammatory reaction in the body. AITD patients can have *multiple* triggers throughout life! Because of genetic predisposition, the virus or other autoimmune trigger uses various immune signals to make unauthorized changes to the T cell soldier "training manual."

These soldiers-in-training having been sitting around twiddling their thumbs for ages. They haven't been exposed to farm animals or pigpens, and have remained in a largely industrialized, sterile environment. They don't know any better, and are ill-prepared to attack. Confused and naïve, they read the new training manual that now instructs them to mount an attack against the thyroid gland itself. And they proceed!

Many, but not all, Hashimoto's patients can identify a trigger in the time leading up to diagnosis. Think back to the months or even years before you or your loved one started getting sick. Did you have a bad cold?

Mono? A viral infection like the flu or shingles? Did you have a bad allergic reaction? What about a stressful life event? In AITD, there can be many triggers to set off the disease process. Even severe stress can and does often trigger autoimmunity! Listed below are commonly cited triggers, but there are probably many others that haven't yet been described.

TABLE 3.2. HASHIMOTO'S TRIGGERS

INFECTIONS

Viral Infections	Influenza virus	Lyme Disease
Adenovirus	Measles/Mumps/Rubella	Rickettsia
Coxsackievirus (Hand-Foot-and-Mouth Disease)	Parvovirus B19 (childhood rash)	Yersinia enterocolitica (bacterial infection of the gut contracted from foods)
CMV	Retroviruses (HTLV-1, HFV, HIV, SV40)	
EBV (mononucleosis)	VZV (Chicken Pox/Shingles)	**Fungal Infections**
Enterovirus (stomach bug)	**Bacterial Infections**	Candida Albicans (yeast infection)
Herpes Simplex Virus (including HHV-6)	Coxiella burnetii	**Parasites**
Hepatitis C or B	H. Pylori (an infection of the stomach that increases risk for stomach ulcers)	Blastocystis hominis

DRUGS, TOXINS, AND ALLERGENS

Environmental toxins	Immunotherapies (such as certain chemotherapy drugs or medications for other autoimmune disease)	Severe allergic reaction to medications (such as antibiotics)
Food allergies or sensitivities (most commonly, gluten, dairy, soy, nuts, and corn)		Severe seasonal allergies

STRESSFUL LIFE EVENTS

Pregnancy and giving birth	Severe illness	Trauma
Hospitalization	Stressful life events like divorce, family death, job loss, or moving	
Surgery		

STEP THREE: A Sustained Autoimmune Response

Some people's soldiers-in-training receive a training manual with a couple pages missing, while others receive a completely different manual instructing widespread self-destruction. That is to say, some autoimmune responses are mild and others are more severe. It all depends on your specific trigger and how your individual immune system responds. Mild responses are much more likely to go into disease remission, where the immune system gets back on track and stops attacking the thyroid gland. More on disease remission in Chapter 12.

If you can quiet your immune system and get it back on track before it completely destroys the gland, you may avoid future effects of hypothyroidism and other autoimmune diseases. But this is no easy task! It involves working with a qualified doctor to uncover your autoimmune trigger(s) and minimize continued misdirection to your immune system. Redirecting the immune system is patient-specific. *There is no one-size-fits-all approach.*

With Graves' disease, 30 percent of patients can go into remission. With Hashimoto's disease, it is typically more challenging and difficult. In both diseases, there may be times when you are in remission, and times when you start again with active disease—this is normal! We will discuss various vitamins, diets, medical treatments, and how to avoid immune triggers while fighting for remission in upcoming chapters.

HASHIMOTO'S ANTIBODIES

When talking about Hashimoto's disease, it is important that we review the different antibodies produced by the immune system that signal an attack on the thyroid gland. As discussed in the last chapter, B cells are snipers that shoot off different types of bullets (or antibodies) targeting important machinery at the thyroid factory. The antibodies themselves don't destroy the machines; instead, they are signals to the foot soldiers (or the T cells) to attack and kill the thyroid cells. The more antibodies in your blood, the more active your immune system is against your thyroid gland. Reducing Hashimoto's antibodies is one of our primary goals in disease management. We will discuss this in more detail in Part 3.

Thyroid Peroxidase Antibodies

Thyroid Peroxidase Antibodies (TPOAbs) are the most common antibodies in Hashimoto's disease. TPOAbs are bullets targeted against the first step of thyroid hormone production: the uptake of iodide in the diet to form thyroid hormone. When present, they signal T cells to go to hand-to-hand combat with thyroid peroxidase, one of your most important thyroid hormone-producing machines.

Thyroglobulin Antibodies

Thyroglobulin Antibodies (TGAbs) are the second most common antibody. These bullets are directed at one of the largest proteins in your body, thyroglobulin. In fact, thyroglobulin makes up 50 percent of your thyroid gland. Think of thyroglobulin as a precursor to T4 and T3. When thyroglobulin attaches to iodine, it gets processed on the thyroid factory conveyor belt to make thyroid hormone.

TSH Receptor Antibodies

TSH Receptor Antibodies (TSHRAbs or TRAbs, for short) are bullets directed at the mailbox where the thyroid cell receives its instructions from the pituitary gland. Usually, TRAbs cause hyperthyroidism, instructing the thyroid cells to make more and more thyroid hormone and eliminating the "off" button. These antibodies are almost always seen in Graves' disease, but may also be seen at a low level in Hashimoto's.

THE MANY FACES OF HASHIMOTO'S

By now you understand that there are many different reasons people get Hashimoto's disease, leading to extensive disease variety. The symptoms you have may be entirely different from the ones others experience. The antibodies you have may be completely different than those patients with the same disease process.

Because of this, we now can identify six different forms of Hashimoto's (although there are probably many more that exist, but are yet to be identified.). The different forms of Hashimoto's can best be determined under the microscope, although an experienced thyroid doctor can diagnose them through medical history, blood work, and imaging. We will look further into the diagnosis and treatment in Part 2.

The different forms of Hashimoto's include:

The Classic Form

This is the most common form of Hashimoto's disease. It is usually diagnosed between ages thirty to sixty, and is overwhelmingly more common in women than men, with a ratio of twelve women for every one man. Up to 75 percent of these patients are initially told that they have normal thyroid labs, despite having many Hashimoto's symptoms. The disease can perpetuate many years of gland destruction before thyroid levels start to enter the established abnormal ranges, at which point patients are typically started on treatment.

The Fibrous/Fibrosing Variant

This is the second most common form of Hashimoto's, but it tends to occur in older women in their sixties and seventies. It usually presents as a goiter, or enlargement of the thyroid gland, and is associated with a lot of scar tissue in and around the thyroid gland. It is more common in women, at a ratio of 10:1.

The IGG4-Related Variant

This variant occurs less often, presenting in the early forties and fifties. It occurs more often in women, with a ratio of three women for one man, but can occur commonly in men. Thyroid antibodies can reach extremely high levels, even into the thousands. The IGG4 form of Hashimoto's disease can be associated with other types of autoimmune diseases, which we will discuss further in the next chapter.

The Juvenile Variant

This form of Hashimoto's happens in teenagers, and like the other forms of Hashimoto's, is more common in females, with a ratio of six women for one man. Typically starting at ages ten to eighteen, kids may complain of neck enlargement or feeling like there is something in their throat. In almost half of cases, teens have normal thyroid levels, with close to half having varying degrees of hypothyroidism. Some may even present in hyperthyroidism and progress to hypothyroidism, or go into remission.

The Hashitoxicosis Variant

This form of Hashimoto's occurs in patients' ages forty to sixty. It is more common in women, at a ratio of five women for one man. Although "hashitoxicosis" is a fancy name for hyperthyroidism, patients with this form of Hashimoto's can have a full spectrum of disease, including severe hyperthyroidism, or toggle back and forth between hypothyroid and hyperthyroid symptoms. Patients can have TSH levels that are low, normal, or slightly high.

The Postpartum Variant

This variant occurs in the twelve months following pregnancy. Some reports have suggested that this can occur in one of every twelve deliveries, but is much more common in women who already have Hashimoto's antibodies. Many times, it is never diagnosed. Two to five months after delivery, the patient can develop hyperthyroidism that lasts for about a month. Following this, the patient can develop hypothyroidism that lasts for about two to six months, and is sometimes confused with postpartum depression. Many times, these patients can go into remission and get back to a normal thyroid state, but this is not always possible.

HASHIMOTO'S THROUGHOUT LIFE

Hashimoto's can affect you at many times in your life. During these life stages, it is important for you to know how AITD can affect other aspects of your health.

Hashimoto's and Fertility

If your thyroid levels are off, you may first notice that your menstrual cycles become irregular. If you are someone who has regular periods like clockwork, you may notice that you have more frequent cycles, or don't get your period for months at a time. You may also notice that your periods become heavier or more painful. In addition, PMS can get worse. AITD can increase your risk of infertility and miscarriage—and that is why it is important to work with your doctor to ensure that your thyroid levels are optimized and your antibodies are decreasing before attempting pregnancy.

Hashimoto's and Pregnancy

If you have AITD and get a positive pregnancy test, contact your doctor immediately for thyroid blood tests. It is important to make sure that you have healthy thyroid levels; this is particularly important in the first ten weeks of gestation, when the fetus doesn't have its own thyroid gland and is relying on your thyroid medicine to grow and develop normally. Also, if you are unaware that you have underlying Hashimoto's, delivery can serve as an autoimmune trigger. After pregnancy, thyroid levels can bounce all over the place—and in these cases, become hyperthyroid, then hypothyroid, and eventually (in many cases), returning to normal. During and after pregnancy, it is important to work with your doctor to ensure your thyroid levels remain normal.

Hashimoto's and Menopause

As if menopause itself is not hard enough, autoimmune thyroid disease can make it even harder. Sometimes, Hashimoto's patients can develop early menopause. Other times, thyroid abnormalities will worsen hot flashes and propel you on an emotional rollercoaster. For all female patients, the changes in your estrogen levels can affect thyroid medication dosing. This is yet another life stage where it is important to aggressively follow and optimize your thyroid levels.

Hashimoto's and Other Medical Conditions

In addition to typical Hashimoto's symptoms, there are other medical diagnoses that can worsen when someone has an underlying thyroid disorder. If you have been diagnosed with one of the following medical conditions, it is a good idea to discuss with your doctor whether your thyroid disorder is impacting your other health issues. As you can see, we weren't kidding when we said that the thyroid gland has effects from the top of your head to the tip of your toes! (See Table 3.3 on page 42.)

TABLE 3.3. CONDITIONS WORSENED BY HYPO OR HYPERTHYROIDISM		
HYPOTHYROIDISM CAN WORSEN...		
Blood pressure (the bottom number)	Decreased kidney function	Obesity
	Depression	Sleep apnea
Bradycardia (low heart rate)	Gallstones	Swelling in your face, legs, and feet
Congestive heart failure	High cholesterol	
HYPERTHYROIDISM CAN WORSEN...		
Anxiety and panic attacks	Blood pressure (the top number)	Insomnia
Atrial fibrillation (fast heart rhythm)	Blood sugar (high or low)	Osteoporosis
	Congestive heart failure	Psychosis or suicidal thoughts
		Tachycardia (high heart rate)

In addition to worsening the above medical conditions, AITD is associated with the development of other autoimmune diseases. It is important to know what these other autoimmune diseases are so that you can be watchful for symptoms. If you continue to have fatigue, for example, even when your thyroid levels are normalized, you may have another underlying autoimmune disease. We will dive further into this in the next chapter.

CONCLUSION

That's a lot to absorb, isn't it? But now you have an understanding of what Hashimoto's is, where it comes from, and its possible effects on your body and health. All of this information can be overwhelming. But remember, as you read the following chapters, you will learn how to deal with Hashimoto's in order to feel better. Before you seek treatment for a medical condition (whether it's with medication or lifestyle changes), you should know as much as you can about the condition itself. You are your own best advocate in your thyroid care! It is therefore important to have a basic understanding of the autoimmune illnesses that may complicate your Hashimoto's diagnosis.

Before we discuss the diagnosis and treatment of Hashimoto's, let's review some of the other autoimmune diseases that commonly occur

with Hashimoto's. In the next chapter, you will develop a deeper understanding of how your genes contribute to autoimmunity. You will learn
how autoimmune symptoms are different (or in some cases, remarkably
similar!) so that you can distinguish whether your ongoing symptoms
are Hashimoto's-related or possibly attributable to another form of autoimmune disease.

4.

Hashimoto's Thyroiditis and Other Autoimmune Diseases

In the last chapter, we learned that your inherited gene set can play a role in the development of AITD. We will now learn that that same gene set can be responsible for the development of a variety of additional auto-immune diseases.

Before we begin, it is important to know that approximately 75 percent of people with Hashimoto's disease do not have any other autoimmune disease. That leaves 25 percent who do or will. It is therefore vital to arm yourself with information on what other symptoms and conditions to look for in case you do develop another autoimmune disease. This chapter will explore the autoimmune illnesses commonly found in patients who also have Hashimoto's thyroiditis. This includes:

- Autoimmune hives

- Autoimmune polyglandular syndrome (APGS)

- Celiac disease

- Chronic fatigue syndrome (CFS)

- Fibromyalgia

- Inflammatory bowel disease (IBD)

- Multiple sclerosis (MS)

- Postural tachycardia syndrome (POTS)

- Rheumatoid arthritis

- Systemic lupus erythematosus (SLE)

- Type 1 diabetes mellitus

- Vitiligo

AUTOIMMUNE GENES AND HASHIMOTO'S

One in four people with Hashimoto's disease will develop another auto-immune disease at some point in their lives. While that is a significant number, it means you have a 75 percent chance of never receiving another autoimmune diagnosis. Even though the odds are in your favor, it is important to educate yourself on the other autoimmune diseases that are commonly associated with Hashimoto's.

There are different ways that Hashimoto's can occur with other autoimmune diseases. Sometimes, several members of a family have different autoimmune diseases. This is called *familial autoimmunity*. Other times, one member of a family has more than one autoimmune disease. The term for this is *polyautoimmunity* (meaning more than one autoimmune disease in the same person). When an individual has more than three autoimmune diseases, we refer to that as *multiple autoimmune syndrome* (MAS), or *autoimmune polyglandular syndrome* (APGS, for short). Don't be overly concerned about the technical names—what's important to understand is that autoimmune disease can have a genetic component. In the following sections, we will explore the various forms of autoimmunity that can occur in Hashimoto's patients.

Know Your Family Tree

Most of us are not really aware of our family's medical history. We might know about our parents' and our grandparents' health, but that's where it ends. Many times, because of societal norms, embarrassment, or just plain forgetfulness, we don't adequately equip ourselves with the information we need to understand our genetic predispositions.

Your family history can tell you a lot about your risk for developing high blood pressure, heart disease, cancer, and, not surprisingly, autoimmune disease. So the next time you are at a family gathering, get out a piece of paper and collect your family's medical history to the best of your ability. Don't be afraid to ask questions. Mapping out your family's medical history can help you to identify the autoimmune diseases you may be at risk for developing in the future. And just as important, it can be helpful to your relatives, including future generations, yet to be born.

Back to Your Genes

In the last chapter, we discussed Hashimoto's-specific genes in the development of Hashimoto's and inheriting one of two gene sets. The first gene set is thyroid-specific and probably plays a minor role in disease development. The second gene set is immune-specific and will be the focus of our discussion.

There are many different genes involved in the immune system. These genes are the instructions in the T cell soldier training manual directing them to remain quiet or mount an attack. The specific gene set that you were born with is not only important in development of Hashimoto's, but can instruct your T cells to attack a variety of other tissues in your body, leading to other forms of autoimmune disease.

In Figure 4.1, we have listed some of the more common family gene sets and associated autoimmune illnesses. If you have taken your family medical history, place a checkmark next to the diseases that run in your family. If you can't identify a family member with any other autoimmune disease, great! This suggests that you may never develop another form of autoimmunity. Remember, it is much more common to have Hashimoto's disease as your one and only autoimmune illness.

Several common autoimmune family gene sets are shown in the graphic on the following page. Each gene set lists the autoimmune diseases found in families with that particular gene. Genetic issues are extremely complex and technical, and a detailed scientific explanation would be beyond the scope of this book. However, we do want you to understand which autoimmune diseases fall into certain genetic categories. Although we've included the scientific name for each gene set, the focus in the figure is on the groupings of particular diseases along with their genetic connection.

As you can see, several autoimmune illnesses are listed multiple times under different gene sets. In fact, autoimmune thyroid disease is common among all of them. Multiple sclerosis, lupus, type 1 diabetes, celiac disease, rheumatoid arthritis, and myasthenia gravis also occur in more than one gene set associated with familial autoimmunity. You may have checked off diseases that are listed multiple times in different categories, but you may also have narrowed it down to two or three different candidate genes. Your family assessment will be helpful as we explore autoimmune diseases, allowing you to concentrate on the types of autoimmune diseases that may be more likely to develop in the future.

Looking at this list of autoimmune illnesses can be overwhelming. Its purpose is to raise awareness that many forms of autoimmune disease can occur when you inherit particular gene sets. Development of other forms of autoimmune disease is more likely if you have a strong family history.

It is therefore important to understand what these diseases are and what to look for, as we will learn later in the chapter.

Thyroid Quick Tip: Autoimmune diseases are related and tend to cluster together in families and in individuals.

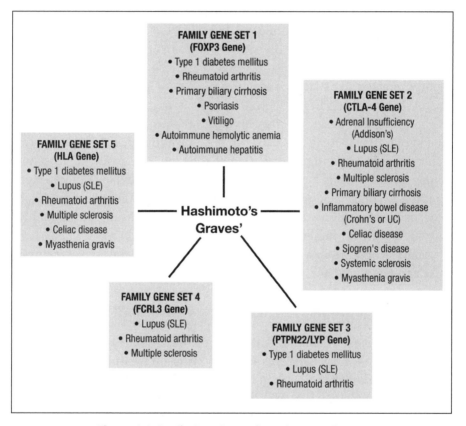

Figure 4.1. Family Gene Sets and Autoimmune Diseases
Source: Dr. Brittany Henderson

FAMILY AUTOIMMUNE DISEASES ASSOCIATED WITH HASHIMOTO'S

Let's explore the most common autoimmune diseases that can occur in families with Hashimoto's disease. If you have Hashimoto's, it's important to be aware of these associated conditions, so if you develop any of them, you can seek treatment as soon as possible. For more information on other autoimmune disorders listed above, see the Resources on page 239.

■ Type 1 Diabetes Mellitus

Of all autoimmune conditions, the familial clustering of AITD and type 1 diabetes is one of the most common. Type 1 diabetes mellitus, also called juvenile diabetes, is a disease that normally shows up in childhood, as opposed to type 2 diabetes, which typically occurs in adults. If you have type 1, you have a 50-percent chance of developing Hashimoto's disease at some point in your life. If you have Hashimoto's, but don't have type 1, it is much less likely that you will develop diabetes—but there is still an increased risk. Despite being a childhood disease, type 1 can also develop in adulthood, usually referred to as latent autoimmune disease of adulthood (LADA).

LADA usually occurs between the ages of twenty-five to fifty-five, with an average age at onset of forty. Similar to the process in Hashimoto's, B cells shoot off pancreas-specific "bullets," or antibodies. Symptoms can include weight loss, fatigue, urinating all the time, and excessive thirst and hunger. Some patients have no presenting symptoms and high blood sugar is picked up on screening blood work. Type 1 and LADA are more likely to occur if autoimmune disease runs on your father's side of the family, particularly if your father has T1DM himself.

Many people are able to manage their diabetes with the help of their primary care physician, while others are under the care of an endocrinologist.

■ Rheumatoid Arthritis

First and foremost, rheumatoid arthritis, or RA, is not the same disease as old-age arthritis or osteoarthritis. Osteoarthritis is a wearing down of joints and is much more common than RA. Osteoarthritis is *not* an autoimmune disease. Conversely, RA *is* an autoimmune disease, aimed at particular joints in the body associated with inflammation, resulting in swelling, redness, and stiffness in the morning when waking. Joints typically involved include the hands, the wrists, and the feet. If you or a loved one has Hashimoto's, you have an increased chance of having someone in your family with rheumatoid arthritis. If you have rheumatoid arthritis, it's best to be under the care of a rheumatologist.

■ Systemic Lupus Erythematosus (SLE)

Because there is symptom overlap between Hashimoto's disease and lupus, it is extremely common for patients to test positively on an ANA (antinuclear antibody) blood test, which is typically used to screen for SLE (systemic lupus erythmatosus).

In some reports, the likelihood of having a positive ANA test in Hashimoto's is upwards of 70 percent. But having a positive ANA doesn't necessarily mean you have lupus! In most cases, the overactive immune system in Hashimoto's disease can cause a falsely positive ANA test. Still, it can sometimes indicate another autoimmune disease and, if you have a positive ANA, you should discuss it with your doctor.

Lupus is a systemic disease, meaning that it can cause issues all over the body. Common symptoms to look for include extreme fatigue (this is also the most common symptoms in Hashimoto's), joint pain, a rash on the cheeks and nose, anemia (low blood cell count), unexplained fever, and other issues with the kidney and blood vessels. Some studies have reported that up to one in five patients with lupus have positive Hashimoto's antibodies (even if they have normal thyroid levels), with one in eight lupus patients developing full blown AITD. Because symptoms overlap with a variety of other illnesses, it is important to work with both your primary doctor and rheumatologist to help understand and manage lupus.

Sjogren's Disease and Systemic Sclerosis

Sjogren's disease and systemic sclerosis are two additional diseases related to lupus. Sjogren's disease typically manifests as excessive dry mouth and dry eyes and is relatively common in patients with Hashimoto's. Systemic sclerosis (sometimes called scleroderma) is an autoimmune disease that causes skin thickening on the hands, feet, and face. More severe forms of systemic sclerosis can cause stiffness to all organs in the body, contributing to organ failure. Like lupus, a rheumatologist can help manage both conditions.

■ Multiple Sclerosis (MS)

Multiple sclerosis (MS) is an autoimmune disease of the nervous system. The immune system typically attacks the protective layer surrounding your nerve cells called myelin in the brain and spinal cord. MS occurs more often in the Northern Hemisphere (farther from the equator), likely due to clustering of people from certain genetic backgrounds and specific regional autoimmune triggers. People with MS have Hashimoto's disease ten times more frequently than those who don't. If you have MS, make sure you work with a neurologist to best manage your symptoms.

■ Celiac Disease

You've probably heard of gluten intolerance and celiac disease, due to all the attention they have received in the media and all over the Internet. Celiac disease is an autoimmune disease of the small intestine after exposure to gluten, a wheat protein found in many breads and grains. One in twenty people with Hashimoto's disease also have celiac disease. Celiac disease is much more common in people of Northern European descent, particularly Irish. Symptoms include abdominal bloating, gas, and diarrhea. Avoiding gluten in the diet can treat the disease. Because the media has popularized celiac disease, Hashimoto's patients commonly wonder if they should follow a gluten-free diet. There is no universal "yes" or "no" to this question. It depends, and this is something we will address in detail in Chapter 9. If you have celiac disease, a gastroenterologist can help to best manage your symptoms.

■ Inflammatory Bowel Disease (IBD)

Inflammatory bowel disease (IBD) includes both Crohn's disease and ulcerative colitis and is an autoimmune disease of the intestine. Ulcerative colitis causes inflammation of the large intestine, while Crohn's disease causes inflammation of the complete digestive tract. Both forms of IBD can present with blood in the stool and persistent diarrhea. Early treatment of Hashimoto's disease in IBD is important, because thyroid dysfunction can worsen bowel symptoms. If you have either form of IBD, it's important to be under the care of a gastroenterologist.

■ Vitiligo

Vitiligo is an autoimmune disease of the skin cells causing loss of pigment (color) in the skin. As a result, people can get patches of lighter skin on their hands, face, and chest. In some people, the patches don't grow in size, but in others, the patches can expand. Sometimes this happens slowly, and other times it occurs at a fast pace. Although vitiligo is difficult to treat, some success has been found with topical steroids and ultraviolet therapy. Since dermatologists specialize in diseases of the skin, they are the best type of doctor to see if you have been diagnosed with vitiligo or believe you have it. One in five patients with vitiligo also have Hashimoto's thyroiditis.

As you can see, many autoimmune diseases can occur in families and individuals with AITD. Because the immune system can attack multiple organ systems throughout the body, AITD patients oftentimes must work with a variety of specialists (including endocrinologists, rheumatologists, gastroenterologists, neurologists, and dermatologists) to manage their disease process. Since we have explored the autoimmune diseases that occur commonly in families with AITD, we will move next to autoimmune diseases that cluster in individual patients.

INDIVIDUAL AUTOIMMUNE DISEASES THAT CAN OCCUR WITH HASHIMOTO'S

In addition to familial autoimmunity, there are some less common gene sets that can result in polyautoimmunity, or multiple autoimmune diseases in the same individual. Individuals with these polyautoimmune-prone gene sets can also get any and all combinations of autoimmune diseases listed in the previous section. When a person is diagnosed with three or more autoimmune illnesses, we refer to this as *multiple autoimmune syndrome* (MAS), or sometimes *autoimmune polyglandular syndrome* (APGS).

There are three commonly described APGS syndromes, although there are likely many other autoimmune syndromes that haven't yet been described. Here we will briefly discuss the types of autoimmune diseases found in individuals with APGS.

■ Autoimmune Polyglandular Syndrome (APGS)

Some individuals with Hashimoto's disease develop a specific combination of autoimmune diseases that can be classified as APGS Type I, II, or III. Type I is rare and usually manifests in childhood, with widespread autoimmunity activity against multiple glands. Type II is characterized by the development of three specific autoimmune diseases, including: autoimmune thyroid disease (AITD), type 1 diabetes mellitus, and adrenal insufficiency (also called Addison's disease). Patients with type II APGS also may develop celiac disease and early menopause (autoimmunity against the ovaries).

Type III APGS is broken down into three subcategories, all with AITD as the main component. In people with Type III APGS, they have AITD and one of the following diseases: Type 1 diabetes mellitus, pernicious anemia (autoimmune vitamin B$_{12}$ deficiency), vitiligo, or alopecia (complete baldness due to an autoimmune attack on the hair follicle). Although there are specific combinations of autoimmune diseases formally recognized as APGS I, II or III, it is important to remember that, in polyautoimmunity, individuals can have any combination of autoimmune illness.

Allison's Experience: Dealing with Hashimoto's and Other Autoimmune Diseases

You know how it is when you constantly don't feel well. There have been times when I've been confined to bed for days, unable to eat, get dressed, or do anything productive or enjoyable.

After having CFS and fibromyalgia for many years, I was later diagnosed with Hashimoto's. In a strange way, it was a relief. While CFS and fibromyalgia are controversial (despite being established as real illnesses), Hashimoto's is not. When the diagnosis came, it was a confirmation that my years of suffering had been related to an autoimmune process, as I has suspected. Over the years, it has felt on a visceral level as if my body was attacking itself.

Once I had a diagnosis, I was able to get treatment. Over time, my Hashimoto's became better controlled. It wasn't quick, and there were times that I doubted if I would ever feel better. Patience is required, and that's not easy when you feel weak and have no energy. But eventually (under Dr. Henderson's care), I did start having an improvement in my symptoms. As time went on, I was surprised to find that the more controlled my Hashimoto's became, the fewer flare-ups I had with my CFS and fibro.

Yes, I still have flare-ups. I still have bad days, and some of those times it's hard to tell which of my autoimmune illnesses are at play. Other times, I can tell the flare-up starts as CFS or fibro, but then also triggers a worsening of my Hashimoto's. When I go through an extended rough patch, I have my thyroid levels tested—and many times, my thyroid medicine needs adjustment. When my thyroid levels improve, so typically do my symptoms.

Interestingly, the same factors affect all of my autoimmune problems. Lack of restorative sleep, stress, deficiencies of certain vitamins and minerals (check out Chapter 10), allergies, and getting any kind of virus/bacterial infection will set off an autoimmune chain reaction (see more on this in Chapter 12). But the good news is that when I (and you) can get one of these under control, the others will typically follow.

OTHER AUTOIMMUNE DISEASES
THAT CAN OCCUR WITH HASHIMOTO'S

In this section, we will touch on other diseases that are commonly seen in patients with Hashimoto's. In many cases, scientists are still working on whether the diseases listed below have an autoimmune origin, how to diagnose them, and how to effectively treat them.

■ Fibromyalgia

Fibromyalgia is a chronic, widespread pain syndrome associated with muscle pain throughout the body, not joint pain. Autoimmune thyroid disease occurs commonly in patients with fibromyalgia. The pain of fibromyalgia and the pain that occurs with Hashimoto's can mimic one another, and are oftentimes hard to differentiate. Although highly debated, some scientists suggest that fibromyalgia, too, has an autoimmune basis. Specifically, fibromyalgia patients may have elevated blood inflammation markers and an immune response against small-fiber nerve endings and pain receptors.

■ Autoimmune Hives

Many times Hashimoto's and Graves' disease patients can develop red, itchy hives on their skin. Hives can develop multiple times a week or even multiple times in a single day. The technical name for these hives is "auto-immune urticaria." People with recurrent hives have thyroid antibodies eight times more commonly than the general population. There are several available treatments, but these types of hives can be very difficult to treat.

■ Postural Tachycardia Syndrome (POTS)

Postural tachycardia syndrome, or POTS, is a condition manifested by heart racing and dizziness. The diagnosis often follows a viral infection and occurs commonly in women. Studies suggest that there may be an autoimmune component. Approximately 30 percent of POTS patients also have Hashimoto's antibodies. In fact, Hashimoto's disease is the most common autoimmune disorder that occurs in POTS. Other autoimmune diseases that can co-occur include: rheumatoid arthritis, lupus (one in four POTS patients have a positive ANA), and immune deficiency syndrome.

■ Chronic Fatigue Syndrome (CFS)

Chronic fatigue syndrome or CFS is a condition characterized by excessive and persistent fatigue limiting a person's ability to carry out ordinary daily tasks. Patients are extremely sensitive to normal amounts of exercise and daily activity. Although fatigue is closely associated with CFS, there are many other symptoms that overlap with Hashimoto's symptoms. These include chills, headaches, sleeping difficulties, body aches, and brain fog. Also, there can be a general feeling of sickness that CFS patients have that is similar to that of Hashimoto's.

Although there is no consensus about the exact cause, patients have been shown to have elevations in inflammation markers, increased oxidative stress in the body, and abnormal mitochondria (think of mitochondria as the engines inside your cells that keep them working). Up to 60 percent of CFS patients have other autoimmune diseases.

CONCLUSION

As you can see, Hashimoto's disease overlaps with many other autoimmune diseases. Symptoms that you had previously attributed to Hashimoto's may, indeed, be from uncontrolled Hashimoto's, or may be stemming from another underlying autoimmune illness. This can be frustrating to Hashimoto's patients, because there isn't a definitive way to determine which autoimmune disease is at work, causing symptoms. When you have more than one autoimmune illness, a flare up of one can trigger any others you have. This is why, it's so important to discuss your symptoms with your doctor.

Now that we have built a foundation for understanding thyroid disease, particularly Hashimoto's, we will look into the testing and diagnosis of AITD.

PART 2

Testing and Diagnosis

5.

Understanding Thyroid Blood Tests

In the first two chapters, we gave an overview of what the most common thyroid lab tests are and why they are measured. But there are many subtle factors to be aware of when trying to understand the results of thyroid blood with regard to thyroid levels. In this chapter, we will explore thyroid lab tests and what tests are (and aren't) most useful. We will also examine how various factors may influence your thyroid levels. Lastly, we will equip you on how to prepare in advance for your thyroid laboratory testing. Because you will need to have thyroid labs checked regularly throughout your lifetime, having a clear understanding of what to be aware of in your lab results will be of vital importance on your thyroid journey.

THE BASICS OF THYROID TESTING

There are many available blood tests to check thyroid function. Many medical providers feel comfortable ordering a thyroid-stimulating hormone (TSH) test or a free thyroxine (free T4) level, but do not routinely order the other labs.

You may be wondering why this is the case. The main reason is that TSH and free T4 are the two most reliable thyroid blood tests. In this section, we will discuss these standard thyroid tests and their normal ranges.

TSH

Arguably, TSH is the most important thyroid blood level. As stated in Chapter 1, TSH is an average reading of how well your thyroid has been working (or not working) over the past month. Remember to think of TSH as the electric meter at your house. Read once a month, it can tell you on average how your thyroid levels have been doing in the past thirty days, but it doesn't tell you how much thyroid hormone you've produced on a daily basis. Thus, TSH is a "bird's eye" view (from the viewpoint of the pituitary gland in your brain) of your body's thyroid supply over time. It doesn't tell you everything, as you will learn, but it's an important piece of the thyroid puzzle.

The TSH Controversy

TSH has gotten a lot of bad press on blogs and social media, with many patients frustrated when their test comes back "normal," even when they're suffering from symptoms of AITD. While this frustration is completely understandable, there are several reasons this may occur. In Chapter 3, when discussing the different forms of Hashimoto's, we mentioned that up to 75 percent of those diagnosed with the classic form may actually have normal thyroid levels at diagnosis. To understand why this occurs, we must address a central question in thyroid care: What constitutes a "normal" TSH?

Currently, the standard laboratory reference range for a normal TSH is 0.5 to 5.5 uIU/ml, or similar, depending on the normal reference range at your laboratory. But how did they decide that 0.5 to 5.5 uIU/ml was normal?

Thyroid Quick Tip: The unit uIU/ml is the typical unit of measurement for TSH. IU stands for "International Unit," or an internationally agreed upon unit of measurement. uIU means one millionth of an IU. The unit "ml" stands for milliliter.

Back in 2002, a national survey called the National Health and Nutrition Examination Survey (NHANES III) looked at TSH levels in 16,533 patients who were considered to be healthy and without thyroid disease. They compiled the data, and reported the "normal" range as that which 95 percent of participants fell into, and, *voila*, that's how we have the current normal reference range. It wasn't until later that they found that many people included as "normal" actually had underlying thyroid dysfunction that artificially increased the normal thyroid range.

When they re-analyzed the data, a reference range of 0.5 to 3 uIU/ml emerged as likely a better indication of "normal." As a result, many of the major endocrine societies, including the American Association for Clinical Endocrinologists (AACE) and the American Thyroid Association (ATA) have subsequently revised their normal TSH ranges, though most laboratories are still listing normal ranges up to 5.5 uIU/ml:

- In 2002, AACE narrowed the normal TSH reference range, lowering the upper end of normal to 3.0 uIU/ml.

- In 2003, the National Academy of Clinical Biochemistry recommended an upper normal limit at 2.5 uIU/ml.

- In 2003, a consensus statement from AACE, ATA and the Endocrine Society recommended a target TSH of 1.5 uIU/ml for patients on thyroid medicine.

- The 2009 and 2015 ATA guidelines for thyroid cancer patients listed 2.0 uIU/ml as the upper end of normal in low risk patients.

- The 2011 ATA guidelines for hypothyroidism in pregnancy list 2.5 uIU/ml and 3.0 uIU/ml as the upper end of normal in the first trimester and second/third trimesters, respectively.

As you can see, there is a lot of controversy as to what constitutes a normal TSH level, with many leading societies now acknowledging that the normal range should be narrowed. Still, many physicians continue to use the published laboratory reference range as "normal." For the purposes of this book, we will refer to a normal TSH reference range as 0.5 to 3.0 uIU/ml, with target TSH of 1.5 uIU/ml in *most* healthy patients on thyroid medicine. In patients over the age of seventy and in patients with multiple medical conditions (particularly heart issues), your treating physician may target a slightly higher TSH; this will be discussed further in the following sections.

Why Is My TSH Normal if I Have Hashimoto's Symptoms?

Ah, the age-old question! As stated above, TSH is an extremely useful "snapshot" of how your thyroid has been doing over time. As we mentioned, there are situations where people experience Hashimoto's symptoms, despite having what is considered technically "normal" TSH levels. Using two different examples, we'll explain how TSH could look normal in a person who has underlying Hashimoto's disease,

Scenario 1

Mrs. Jones has a TSH of 2.2 uIU/ml. Let's say there was (although there currently isn't) a thyroid monitoring system where her doctor could check her T4 and T3 levels around the clock. At the end of a month, results show that her T4 and T3 in the blood are exactly the same Monday through Sunday and perfectly within the normal range all month long. In this scenario, her TSH reflects normal and consistent thyroid levels. Her TSH, therefore, is normal.

Scenario 2

Mrs. Jones has a TSH of 2.2 uIU/ml and monitors her T4 and T3 for a month, just as in the previous scenario. This time, her T3 and T4 levels are at the higher end of the range on both Monday and Tuesday, but are slightly below the normal range Wednesday through Sunday. On the days her thyroid hormones are below normal, she has less energy and can barely pull herself out of bed. In this scenario, thyroid monitoring reveals Mrs. Jones' inconsistent thyroid levels that have started to become abnormal (hypothyroid), and she is beginning to show signs of Hashimoto's. Despite this, her average monthly reading remains technically within the normal range.

The above scenarios illustrate that it is important to interpret the TSH (which you can think of as an average monthly reading) in the proper context, such as after testing for other thyroid levels, assessing clinical symptoms, and using other diagnostic tests like thyroid ultrasound (see more on this in the next chapter). Always work with your healthcare provider to determine if your levels are normal or abnormal. Additionally, there are many other variables that can affect TSH. We will review them later in the chapter. (See "Thyroid Testing Influences" on page 66.)

FREE T4

Because T4 is the body's bank reserve of thyroid hormone, and because 80 percent of thyroid hormone produced by the thyroid gland is T4, free T4 levels usually remain consistent with time. If your thyroid gland or replacement medicine is working normally, the hormones you take out of your thyroid bank to keep your body functioning should be continuously replenished. A normal free T4 level is usually close to the middle of the normal range, with a typical normal range of 0.6 to 1.4 ng/dl. (Each lab is different, so make sure you always look at your specific normal range.)

The exception to this is in pregnancy, where doctors strive to keep the T4 at the higher end of the normal range, because T4 helps the fetus grow and develop normally. There are various medications and illnesses that can affect your free T4 blood test, which we will explore further later in the chapter.

When you look at your own thyroid blood tests, your free T4 level should remain relatively consistent and stable with time. Keeping your T4 bank full is one of the most important ways to ensure your muscle, liver, brain, and other tissues are seeing enough T3, or active thyroid hormone.

ADDITIONAL THYROID TESTING

There are several additional thyroid tests that are routinely discussed among doctors and patients in the thyroid community: free T3, reverse T3, the free T3/reverse T3 ratio, and total thyroid levels. Here we will discuss each test in detail and review its usefulness in routine laboratory assessment.

Free T3

You now know that T3 is the active form of thyroid hormone. When thyroid hormone "checkpoints"—including deiodinase enzymes (DIO), the pituitary gland, and the thyroid gland—are all working normally, T3 in the blood and tissues fluctuate as needed for proper bodily function. A normal T3 level can fluctuate with time, but in most cases we refer to "normal" as the exact middle of the published normal reference range (for example, 3 pg/ml is normal if the reference range is 2 to 4 pg/ml). Levels towards the bottom or top of the normal range (although technically normal), can still be too low or too high for an individual person, prompting T3 symptoms (keep reading!).

For example, a free T3 level of 3.8 pg/ml, although technically within the normal range of 2 to 4 pg/ml, is at the top end of the range and may be associated with hyperthyroid or high T3 symptoms. It is important to know that, although we have a standardized normal range, everyone has an individualized "normal" T3 set-point that typically falls within this range. Everyone is different.

As said in Chapter 1, the body knows when it needs active thyroid hormone and regulates it quite efficiently in the normal state. When a person is running a marathon, for example, the muscles use T3 as energy, but purposefully decrease T3 after the race to assist in muscle repair and recovery. The same exact scenario happens in someone who has had a heart attack, with T3 decreasing to allow the heart time to slow down and heal. T3 regulation is one of the most important parts of thyroid hormone signaling.

Unfortunately, in Hashimoto's, many of the thyroid hormone "checkpoints" are not working properly. As a result, patients may have what we will call "T3 symptoms," or an imbalance of T3 in the body. Many times, T3 symptoms can result from being on too much (or too little) thyroid replacement medicine (for example, Synthroid and Armour—see Chapter 8). It is important to recognize these symptoms. Below is a list of typical symptoms associated with levels of T3 that are too high or too low.

TABLE 5.1. T3 SYMPTOMS	
Low T3	**High T3**
Brain fog (not thinking clearly)	Anxiety
Cold all the time	Emotional rollercoasters
Depression	Exercise intolerance (out of breath easier)
Fatigue	Fatigue
Gaining weight without diet changes	High heart rate and palpitations
Low heart rate	Hungry all the time (patients also typically gain weight)
Muscle aches	
Sleeping all the time	Shaking (or tremor)
Too tired to exercise	Sweating at night

You'll recognize many of symptoms listed from the hypothyroid and hyperthyroid symptom list in Chapter 3. There is good reason for this, as T3 is the primary driver of these symptoms. Remember that many of these symptoms can also be attributed to other medical conditions unrelated to the thyroid or side effects of medication. Therefore, if you or your loved one has symptoms listed, it is important to discuss them with your doctor.

As you see, *fatigue* is listed in both categories and is the most common T3 symptom. It happens commonly when patients are on either too much or too little thyroid medicine. Are there ways besides a simple T3 blood test and symptoms to figure out how much T3 is inside the cells of your body? Maybe. Researchers are still working on this question, but in the following sections, we will discuss several additional tests that may be of use.

Reverse T3

Many patients have been told that they need a reverse T3 test. You can think of reverse T3 as the opposite of T3, although technically it is derived from breakdown of T4. Remember your deiodinase enzymes (DIO)? When your body is sick or needs to heal itself (for example, after a marathon or heart attack), certain tissues in the body purposefully increase DIO to shunt T4 towards reverse T3 (inactive thyroid derivative—think of this as a blocker of T3), instead of towards active T3. The body does this on purpose in order to give your tissues time to heal.

If the body failed to do this correctly, the injured tissues would see too much active thyroid hormone and scar, instead of take time to heal and repair properly. Some patients become overly concerned with testing and adjusting the reverse T3 value. Instead, the focus should be on optimizing DIO function and reducing inflammation/injury in the body.

Here are some select cases where a reverse T3 blood test may be of value:

- Any severe inflammatory condition (as in rheumatoid arthritis or osteoarthritis)

- Congestive heart failure or heart attack

- Diabetes mellitus Type 2

- End stage kidney disease

- End stage liver disease or cirrhosis

- Hospitalized or acutely ill patients

- Obesity

- Rapid weight loss or anorexia nervosa

- Certain medications (ask your doctor)

In these conditions, checking a reverse T3 may be helpful, but if you are otherwise healthy, the reverse T3 level will come back in the normal range 99 percent of the time. Many integrative medicine practitioners will use reverse T3 in a "free T3 to reverse T3 ratio" to help in thyroid medication dosing.

Free T3/Reverse T3 Ratio

There is some evidence that checking both the free T3 and the reverse T3 may be more helpful than a reverse T3 alone in determining whether the cells of your body are seeing enough T3. Most practitioners state that this ratio should be more than 2:1, with some believing it should be more than 3:1. This means that the active thyroid level should be two to three times that of the inactive thyroid level. But remember, if the DIO "checkpoint" is working correctly, this ratio may be your body's way of telling you that there is an injured tissue or excess inflammation somewhere in the body that needs time to heal.

Instead of throwing more and more T3 into your thyroid regimen, it is important to focus on decreasing inflammation, replacing missing nutrients, and optimizing DIO function. We will discuss this further in Chapters 9 and 10.

TOTAL T3 AND TOTAL T4

In the previous sections and chapters, we have focused on free levels of T4 and T3. This is for good reason—both free T4 and free T3 are more accurate representations of the body's available thyroid hormone. Total T4 and Total T3 can be influenced by alterations in a blood protein called thyroid binding globulin (TBG). Think of TBG as an army of "inflatable rafts" that T4 and T3 attach onto, riding through the bloodstream. When attached to TBG, T4 and T3 are not as readily available to cells. Conversely, since free T4 and free T3 levels are not attached to TBG, they are immediately available to the body.

If TBG rafts are increased or decreased in the blood, total thyroid labs can be artificially high or low. TBG can increase with pregnancy, liver disease, and in patients on birth control pills. Even hypothyroidism itself can increase TBG. TBG can decrease in hyperthyroidism, kidney and liver disease, and with many medications. Additionally, there are several other thyroid transport "rafts," called transthyretin and albumin, that can affect total thyroid levels. Therefore, with few exceptions, many thyroid doctors prefer to check free thyroid levels.

OUTDATED THYROID TESTS

There are several older thyroid tests that are no longer routinely ordered, though some laboratories still have them as part of their thyroid panels. Although not commonly done, we've included them here—in case you've had them done as part of your thyroid testing.

T3 Uptake

This is an indirect measurement of TBG. Factors that alter TBG and total thyroid levels will also artificially increase or decrease T3 uptake. Because we can now measure free thyroid levels and even TBG itself in the blood, the T3 uptake test is no longer the test of choice.

Free Thyroxine Index (FTI)

The free thyroxine index is an indirect measurement of free T4. This test uses Total T4 and the T3 uptake to estimate free levels of T4. We have largely replaced this indirect test with direct testing of free T4.

TESTING SPECIFICALLY FOR AITD

In Chapter 3, we introduced the three main types of antibodies in AITD: thyroid peroxidase antibodies (TPOAbs), thyroglobulin antibodies (TgAbs), and TSH receptor antibodies (TSHRAbs or TRAbs). When testing for Hashimoto's, your doctor may check any or all of these based on whether you have a more hypothyroid or hyperthyroid Hashimoto's signature. In addition to the three main types of antibodies, there are two additional tests that can be performed to measure antibodies in AITD: TSI and TBII.

TSI and TBII

TSI stands for "thyroid-*stimulating* immunoglobulin," whereas TBII stands for "thyroid-binding *inhibitor* immunoglobulin." These two blood tests check whether you have antibodies in your blood that are *stimulating* the thyroid factory to make thyroid hormone or *blocking (inhibiting)* the thyroid from making thyroid hormone. And guess what? You can have both signals at the same time. If you have more stimulating antibodies floating around, you will have more hyperthyroid symptoms. If you have a greater proportion of blocking antibodies, you will have more hypothyroid symptoms. One in five people with Hashimoto's will have TBII blocking antibodies, whereas a smaller proportion will have TSI stimulating antibodies.

The rest simply have TPO, Tg, or TSHR antibodies, or a combination of the three. You should work with your thyroid doctor to determine which of the AITD antibodies are most important for determining your Hashimoto's signature.

THYROID TESTING INFLUENCES

Now that we have reviewed the different thyroid tests, what they mean, and when they are used, there are important nuances that are vital to thyroid lab interpretation. In Chapter 1, we discussed how to determine your thyroid pattern, but, unfortunately, this is not always straightforward. There are other factors to consider when interpreting your thyroid levels. In the next section, we will review many of the factors that can influence your TSH, free T4, and free T3 levels, causing them to change with time.

Age and Your Thyroid

Did you know that TSH is related to age? Studies have shown that the older you get, the higher your TSH goes, normally. There is even scientific data to show that elderly people may actually benefit from a TSH towards the top end of the normal range. In fact, in 2014, the American Thyroid Association raised the target TSH to 4 to 6 uIU/mL in hypothyroid individuals seventy and older. There are a couple of possible reasons for this.

One theory is that older people with multiple medical conditions may have more inflammation and disease in the body, resulting in a mixed signal to the pituitary and causing a slight increase in TSH. Another theory is that TSH elevation with age could reflect undiagnosed thyroid dysfunction. Many studies have shown that the incidence of Hashimoto's disease increases with age, so whether the elevation in TSH in elderly is simply due to underlying undiagnosed AITD is still to be determined.

In a patient with normal T3 and T4 and no symptoms, a TSH level in the 4 to 6 uIU/mL range can be classified as *subclinical hypothyroidism*. In younger patients under the age of sixty-five, untreated subclinical hypothyroidism has been associated with increased risk of death from heart problems, whereas older patients over age sixty-five have shown no signs of increased risk of cardiovascular death in this TSH range. So, for younger patients, treating an elevated TSH in this range makes sense. In young, healthy patients, we like to target a TSH level between 0.5 to 3 uIU/mL—and the closer to 1.5 uIU/mL, the better!

However, if you are over sixty years of age and have no thyroid symptoms, your doctor may elect to closely monitor a TSH level in the 4 to 6 uIU/mL range, rather than treat it. Unfortunately, our current TSH normal range includes all ages and is not broken down into age-appropriate reference ranges.

Below are the median normal TSH levels (the level that a majority of healthy people were at) according to one study based on age. As you can see, with increasing age, normal TSH levels also increase.

TABLE 5.2. TSH LEVELS ACCORDING TO AGE		
AGE (YEARS)	**MEDIAN TSH LEVEL (mU/L)**	**NORMAL REFERENCE RANGE (mU/L)**
18 to 30	1.67	0.52 to 4.15
31 to 40	1.58	0.51 to 3.98
41 to 50	1.65	0.54 to 4.15
51 to 60	1.72	0.51 to 4.36
61 to 70	1.77	0.48 to 4.59
71 to 80	1.82	0.40 to 4.96
81 to 90	1.81	0.36 to 5.49
Over 90	1.86	0.31 to 5.94

Adapted from: Table 2. Vadivello T, Donnan PT, Murphy MJ, Leese GP. "Age- and Gender-Specific TSH Reference Intervals in People With No Obvious Thyroid Disease in Tayside, Scotland: The Thyroid Epidemiology, Audit, and Research Study (TEARS)." *The Journal of Clinical Endocrinology & Metabolism*, Volume 98, Issue 3, 2013.

Gender and Your Thyroid

TSH levels can also be different among men and women. In fact, research shows that women have a slightly higher normal TSH level than men. Since AITD is much more common in women, it is possible that this finding is due to underlying undiagnosed thyroid disease in women, though this is yet to be proven.

Ethnicity and Your Thyroid

Normal TSH can also vary among different ethnicities. Caucasians have the highest TSH levels (median TSH 1.57 uIU/ml), followed by Mexican Americans (median TSH 1.43 uIU/ml), Asian Americans (1.3 uIU/ml), and African Americans (median TSH 1.18 uIU/ml). Studies on other ethnic groups have not yet been done.

Time of Day and Your Thyroid

One of the most important things that can influence your thyroid blood tests is the time of day they are tested. Did you know that many hormones in your body, specifically thyroid hormones, follow a daily rhythm? Take a look at Figure 5.1. TSH levels are highest in the early morning (2 to 4 AM) and lowest in the mid-afternoon (4 PM). The same exact thing goes for free T3. Free T4, on the other hand, is pretty stable with time of day without daily rhythm.

It's important to get labs checked at the same time of day, ideally in the morning! Time of day can alter results to the point where it can be the difference between your doctor starting you on thyroid medicine now, or continuing to needlessly suffer with hypothyroid symptoms without treatment for months or years, while having laboratory tests that appear normal. Time of day can also influence whether your thyroid dosing changes (or doesn't change) based on what your blood results show.

> *Thyroid Quick Tip:* As a rule of thumb, always try to get your thyroid blood tests at the same time of day—ideally first thing in the morning!

Seasons and Your Thyroid

Have you ever heard of seasonal affective disorder (SAD)? SAD encompasses a feeling of sadness and despair that some people get with the

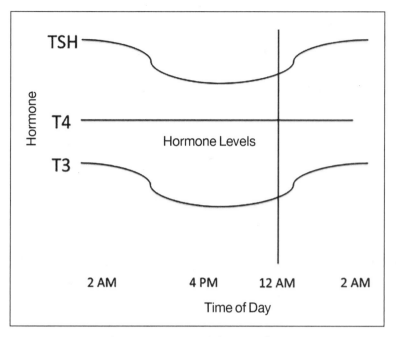

Figure 5.1. TSH Levels by Time of Day

changing seasons, which is worse in the winter. Although there isn't a scientific consensus yet about thyroid dysfunction being linked to SAD, there *is* strong evidence that seasons *do* affect your thyroid blood tests.

In the Yakut people of northeastern Siberia, for example, TSH increases and T4 and T3 levels decrease when going from summer to winter. This has also been shown in other human populations, with TSH significantly rising in winter. This same effect occurs with hibernating bears. We don't know for sure why this happens in humans, but it could have evolutionary roots. "Winter hypothyroidism" may be related to when our human ancestors needed to conserve energy during wintertime months, due to scarcity of crops and food supplies. Therefore, you may notice fluctuations in your thyroid labs as seasons change.

Interfering Medications and Thyroid Hormone

There are multiple medications that affect thyroid laboratory testing. These include prescription medications, over-the-counter vitamins, and supplements. In fact, the FDA recently issued a warning that biotin can cause falsely high or low thyroid blood tests. While we will explore supplements and vitamins extensively in Chapter 10, it is important to know that you should not take biotin vitamins (including multivitamins that contain biotin) and other unnecessary vitamin supplements for forty-eight hours prior to laboratory testing to ensure that you get an accurate test result.

Preparing for Your Thyroid Laboratory Testing

There are certain factors that can affect your thyroid lab test results. Below are some tips to ensure that you get the most accurate results.

- Stop interfering vitamins like biotin (and any other unnecessary vitamins or supplements) forty-eight hours before testing. High-dose biotin treatment (over 5,000 mcg) should be withheld for one to two weeks prior to testing. Do not withhold prescription medicines unless your doctor directs you to do so.

- On the morning of your testing, take your thyroid medicine as you normally would. Do not skip or hold doses prior to testing.

- Have breakfast in the morning as you normally would.

- Thyroid levels should be checked at the same time of day every time they are checked, preferably in the morning.

- Ideally, labs should be drawn two to four hours after thyroid dosing, if thyroid medicines are taken in the morning.

- Your doctor may elect to check both morning thyroid levels and afternoon thyroid levels if your energy levels change throughout the day or week to determine the degree of fluctuation in your TSH and free T3 throughout the day.

On the following pages we have listed a number of common prescription medications that interfere with thyroid levels and alter thyroid metabolism. If you or a loved one is taking one of these medicines, talk to your doctor about potential effects on your thyroid health. *Never* stop or alter prescription medications without consent from your doctor.

TABLE 5.3. PRESCRIPTION MEDICATIONS THAT CAN INFLUENCE THYROID HORMONES

MEDICATION	USED FOR
Amiodarone	Heart conditions like atrial fibrillation
Amphetamines (Vyvanse, Ritalin, Adderall, Phentermine)	ADHD, Weight loss
Anti-seizure medicines (phenobarbital, carbamazepine)	Seizure medications
Aspirin	Blood thinner
Beta blockers (propranolol, metoprolol, atenolol)	Blood pressure and heart rate control
Bile acid sequestrants (cholestyramine, colesevelam, and colestipol)	Cholesterol lowering medicines
Bromocriptine	Pituitary medicine
Cancer therapies (Ipilimumab, Nivolumab, Octreotide, Pembrolizumab, Sunitinib, Sorafenib, Lenvatinib, α-Interferon, 5-FU)	Cancer therapy
Cimetidine (Tagamet)	Anti-stomach ulcer treatment
Diuretics (Acetazolamide, Lasix)	Fluid pills
Estrogens and estrogen disruptors (including Femara, Clomid, Tamoxifen, and Raloxifene)	Birth control pills, hormone replacement therapy in menopause, breast cancer treatment, fertility treatment
Glucocorticoids (steroid medications like prednisone)	Anti-inflammatory, Immunosuppressants
Haldol	Psychiatric drug, anxiety drug
Heparin	Blood thinner
Iodinated contrast (CT scans performed within 6 to 8 weeks of thyroid testing can affect thyroid labs)	Radiology-testing material
Ketoconazole	Antifungal agent
Levodopa	Parkinson's disease
Lithium	Mood stabilizer, bipolar disorder
Metformin	Diabetes medicine
Methimazole (Tapazole)	Graves' disease, hyperthyroidism
NSAIDs	Pain medicine

MEDICATION	USED FOR
Opiates (morphine and derivatives)	Pain medicine
Phosphate Binders (lanthanum carbonate), sevelemer	Phosphate binder in kidney disease
Propylthiouracil (PTU)	Graves' disease, Hyperthyroidism
Reglan (Metoclopramide)	Nausea medication, Gastroparesis medicine
Spironolactone	PCOS medicine, Blood pressure medicine
Sucralfate	Anti-stomach ulcer therapy

Although this list is extensive, there are likely many more prescription medications and herbs/vitamins/supplements that can influence thyroid levels. Therefore, it is important to be selective in the supplements you elect to take, as they all can influence your thyroid "checkpoints" (some positively, others negatively). We will discuss this further in Chapter 10.

Thyroid Quick Tip: A good rule of thumb is to always discuss new medications and vitamins with your thyroid doctor.

These days, most patients can view their test results electronically, through a patient portal. The results always show your number(s), along with the range used at the lab. If you don't use a patient portal to access your results, it's a good idea to ask your doctor to send you a hard copy. This way, you always have your records at your fingertips.

CONCLUSION

Now you understand how involved and intricate thyroid blood testing can be. Unfortunately, it's not as simple as having a basic blood test where the results can be easily interpreted and applied to your treatment plan. It's important to make sure you're getting the specific tests that can help optimize your thyroid health. Many factors affect these tests, including age, ethnicity, gender, time of day, time of year, pre-existing non thyroid medical conditions, and medications/supplements. Being aware of these considerations will help you in assessing what tests may be appropriate for you, and factors that could influence the results.

6.

The Role of Thyroid Imaging

In the previous chapters, we learned what Hashimoto's disease is and the blood tests that can help diagnose it. We also learned that laboratory tests don't always give a clear picture of what's going on with the thyroid—since your TSH can be normal at diagnosis. So what other tests are available to help diagnose you with AITD and other thyroid diseases? In this chapter, we will explore the radiology tests commonly used in thyroid disease. Because many Hashimoto's patients will encounter one or more of these radiology tests in their thyroid journey, it is important to have information on what the tests are, how to prepare for them, and how they can assist in diagnosis.

THYROID ULTRASOUND

Ultrasound is the technical word for a machine that uses sound waves to look at the thyroid gland. Without going too far back to high school physics (who among us wants to do that?), the ultrasound does this through use of something called a "transducer." The transducer, or probe, is a device placed on the skin at the level of the thyroid gland that can produce and receive sound waves. When the transducer is placed on your skin during a thyroid ultrasound, crystals within the probe move back and forth and make energy. That energy is emitted as high frequency sound waves that travel into the skin and "bounce off" the thyroid gland and surrounding structures. The transducer probe then "picks up" the sound waves that bounce back and translates the pattern into a picture of your thyroid gland. Pretty amazing!

Think of this process similar to saying "hello" on the edge of a canyon and hearing the "hello" echo back at you. In the same way, the ultrasound transducer says "hello" to your thyroid gland, and your thyroid gland says "hello" back! The pattern of sound that comes back can tell us a lot about what is going on with your thyroid gland. Because the ultrasound uses sound waves only, there is no radiation associated with this test. Therefore, it is safe to use in all patients, including pregnant women and children.

Who Needs a Thyroid Ultrasound?

Not everybody with AITD will undergo a thyroid ultrasound to directly visualize the gland. There are several reasons for this, but the most important one is that there needs to be some type of clinical indication (feeling something catching in your throat) or physical exam finding (asymmetry, thyroid enlargement) that prompts an ultrasound to be performed. Some patients are sent for thyroid ultrasound after an abnormality is found on imaging performed for another reason, such as a CT scan of the neck after a motor vehicle accident or MRI of the spine performed for neck pain.

Since Hashimoto's patients are at increased risk for thyroid nodules and thyroid cancer, it is important to discuss with your doctor whether there is any thyroid abnormality felt on physical exam and whether a thyroid ultrasound is warranted. Even so, many Hashimoto's patients have underlying thyroid nodules that may not be easily felt on physical exam, so continuously monitoring the thyroid by self-exam for change or growth is extremely important.

Preparing for a Thyroid Ultrasound

If your doctor orders a thyroid ultrasound, there are several things you need to know before, during, and after the exam. Being prepared for the test can help ensure that you receive and complete the test without issue.

Before the Test

Before the thyroid ultrasound begins, there are two things you must know:

1. **You should know who will be performing your thyroid ultrasound.** Currently, there are thyroid specialists (endocrinologists with special training certification) who perform thyroid ultrasounds in the clinic and can give you immediate feedback on what they are seeing as the exam is being performed. (See Resources, beginning on page 239, to find a thyroid doctor.) Other times, you may be sent to a radiology suite to have the exam performed by a radiology technician. Regardless, an experienced doctor or

technician should always be the one performing the thyroid ultrasound, as findings can be influenced by the person who does the procedure. Also, if you have a thyroid abnormality and need another ultrasound test several months down the road, it is best if the same doctor or technician performs the repeat ultrasound to ensure consistency.

2. **You should know what will be done if a thyroid abnormality is found.** Many times, patients are frustrated because they receive thyroid ultrasound reports on an online patient portal, and have no idea how to interpret the results. If you don't get immediate feedback from your thyroid doctor during the exam, it can take several days to weeks to be able to discuss results with your physician. Additionally, some radiology reports include words like "suspicious" and "concerning for cancer," words that most patients don't want to see while casually flipping through results on their cell phones. Make sure that, before you undergo thyroid ultrasound, you discuss with your doctor what next steps will be if a thyroid nodule or other abnormality is found. Having a plan in place "just in case" is comforting and reassuring for all involved.

The Morning of the Test

On the morning of the test, you can eat and drink. Additionally, you should take all prescribed medications and vitamins as you would normally. When getting dressed, select something lightweight, instead of a turtleneck or bulky sweater. A V-neck shirt or scoop neckline is preferred. Avoid wearing a necklace or long, dangling earrings. If you wear makeup, avoid the use of heavy foundation or concealer to the neck. Do not apply excessive amounts of perfume or cologne to the neck. If you have a long beard, trim hair around the neck or bring a hair tie to be able to move the beard out of the way before the exam.

During the Test

During the test, it is important to remain still. Although your performing thyroid doctor or technician may ask you questions, in between answers it is best to not talk. Because the ultrasound probe gives and receives sound waves, talking can interfere with the picture, particularly when measuring blood flow within the gland. Also, avoid excessive swallowing or heavy breathing during the exam, as these motions can cause the gland to move, making it hard to measure.

After the Test

After the test, try not to worry about your test results. If your thyroid doctor performed your exam, you should already know results and next steps. If not, you should have discussed a preliminary plan with your ordering physician prior to the test being performed. Once the ultrasound is complete, there are no other special instructions or restrictions, and you can go about your day normally.

Possible Ultrasound Findings

There is helpful and important information that can be found from a thyroid ultrasound. First and foremost, it can tell you if your thyroid gland is normal. A normal thyroid gland will look bright white, smooth, and normal in size on an ultrasound exam. If you are getting a thyroid ultrasound, it is possible that an abnormality will be found. Here are several abnormalities typically found by thyroid ultrasound.

A Heterogeneous Gland

Heterogeneous is a fancy way of saying, "the thyroid gland is not bright white and smooth, it has a lot of black holes!" You may see this word on your ultrasound report. A heterogeneous gland is the typical finding in someone with underlying AITD—or thyroiditis. But why do AITD patients have a gland full of holes (sometimes referred to as a "Swiss cheese pattern")? First, the gland isn't *actually* full of holes; it just looks that way by ultrasound. Instead of sound waves bouncing back robustly to create a nice bright white image, the sound waves in AITD bounce off a scarred and inflamed gland. The more scar and inflammation, the less the sound waves bounce back, and the darker the image. Therefore, a Hashimoto's gland is dim, dark, and full of irregular areas that look like holes, indicating higher concentrations of scarring and inflammation.

In addition to producing a thyroid image, the thyroid ultrasound also has the ability to detect blood flow within the thyroid gland. In Hashimoto's disease, blood flow can be low, normal, or high, depending on the specific type of Hashimoto's disease. In Graves' disease, blood flow is usually high. Even with a normal TSH, a heterogeneous gland may be a strong indication of underlying AITD.

A Thyroid Nodule (or Nodules)

A nodule is a circular area within the thyroid gland that can appear distinctly dark or light by ultrasound. Whether the nodule is brighter or darker than the surrounding thyroid tissue depends on if it's filled with extra thyroid cells or with fluid, thereby influencing the strength of the sound wave signal traveling back to the transducer. When filled with fluid, a thyroid nodule is referred to as a *thyroid cyst*. But how does fluid fill up in the thyroid gland, and why do nodules occur?

Think of the thyroid again as a thyroid hormone-producing factory. When the factory is under attack by the T cell soldiers and B cell snipers, the factory workers don't leisurely just keep on working—they run and take cover! The factory stops working smoothly and factory items start to pile up. Similarly, nodules represent a piling up of extra thyroid cells or, in some cases, a piling up of extra fluid within the gland. Nodules happen commonly in AITD, but can also be passed along in families, occur due to vitamin deficiencies, and can develop after exposure to environmental toxins, all causing factory production backup.

As discussed in Chapter 2, thyroid nodules are extremely common, affecting up to 80 percent of the normal population. Thankfully, almost all nodules (95 percent) are not cancerous. If a thyroid nodule is found on your scan, there are several descriptive words you may see on your radiology report. The words can help reassure you that the nodule is likely benign (not cancer), or may suggest that a biopsy needs to be performed. (See Chapter 7.) If you have a more suspicious finding by ultrasound, this doesn't necessarily mean that the nodule is cancerous. Actually, it is still much more likely to be benign—so don't panic! Simply discuss the next steps with your doctor. Table 6.1 presents a list of common descriptive words on an ultrasound report that may suggest that the nodule is benign or suspicious and may need further attention.

TABLE 6.1. DESCRIPTIVE WORDS FOR THYROID NODULES			
BENIGN		**SUSPICIOUS**	
Colloid	Simple Cyst	Vascular (lots of blood flow)	Irregular borders
Comet Tail	Spongiform	Taller-Than-Wide	Calcification

An Abnormal Lymph Node

Sometimes a thyroid ultrasound can reveal additional abnormalities, for example an abnormal lymph node. Like thyroid nodules, most lymph nodes found in the neck are completely normal. They *should* be there and are just doing their job, fighting off infection and reacting to environmental allergens. Sometimes, the ultrasound will note the presence of lymph nodes, but state that they appear abnormal. If an abnormal lymph node is found, you should discuss next steps with your doctor. Many times, this entails a lymph node biopsy, which will be covered in the following chapter.

Additional Findings

In addition to the above abnormalities, the thyroid ultrasound can also pick up issues with the structures surrounding the thyroid gland. Parathyroid glands and other types of neck cysts can sometimes be found. Additionally, blockages in your carotid artery, which travels from your heart to your brain through the neck, can also be seen. If any of these are found, be sure to discuss them with your doctor.

NUCLEAR MEDICINE THYROID UPTAKE AND SCAN

The other major type of radiology test used in AITD is the "thyroid uptake and scan." This test is more likely to be ordered if you have Graves' disease, Hashitoxicosis, or thyroid nodules, or if you alternate between hypothyroid and hyperthyroid symptoms. The thyroid scan uses small amounts of material called radiotracer, a special camera, and a computer to provide information on how well the thyroid workers are bringing in iodide from the blood to make thyroid hormone.

If there is increased thyroid hormone production, and thus hyperthyroidism, the uptake scan will be "hot" or "bright." If production has stopped, uptake will be low. Additionally, the scan can tell us whether thyroid workers on the right side of the gland, for example, are working harder than those on the left, and vice versa. Sometimes we see a nodule full of either hard working or lazy thyroid workers that we label a "hot" nodule or a "cold" nodule, depending on uptake. Regardless, the thyroid scan can tell us a lot about how the gland is functioning.

Preparing for an Uptake Scan

If a thyroid scan is ordered, there are several things you should know to ensure that the test goes smoothly. Most nuclear scans are performed at hospitals or radiology offices, although some thyroid doctors can also do the scans in their offices.

Before the Scan

Tell your doctor if there is a possibility you are pregnant or if you are breastfeeding. Also, if you have had iodinated contrast, for example, for a CT scan, in the months prior to scanning, the uptake scan may be inaccurate. Therefore, it is usually advised that you wait until all contrast material has left the body (at least eight weeks) prior to uptake testing. There are interfering medications that prohibit use of an uptake scan, including amiodarone and methimazole/PTU. Discuss whether you need to stop taking any medications prior to scanning with your doctor. Leave jewelry at home and wear loose, comfortable clothing that allows access to your neckline. (See instructions for ultrasound on page 74.) Each radiology department has different instructions, but usually you are asked to not eat for several hours prior to your exam. In the two to three days leading up to the exam, try to avoid consuming high iodine foods like seafood, seaweed, or kelp.

During the Scan

There are two parts to the thyroid uptake and scan.

Part One

The first part involves swallowing the radiotracer (this radiotracer is used for imaging only and is different than radioactive iodine therapy, which will be discussed in Chapter 13). The radiotracer can either be liquid or in capsule form and usually has no taste. Once swallowed, the radiotracer makes its way from your intestines to your bloodstream and then to the thyroid gland. Therefore, you will usually be instructed to go home and return to the nuclear medicine imaging center about four to six hours after swallowing the radiotracer. During this time, you are not dangerous to others and can go about your day as you normally would. At four to six hours, you may be asked to return for the uptake part of the study (although the four to six hour uptake is not always done). A small hand-held device will be held to your knee or other body part to get a baseline measurement, and then held to your neck. Uptake can be high, normal, or low. The uptake part takes about five minutes to complete.

Part Two

You will be asked to return to the center the next day, approximately twenty-four hours after swallowing the pill. At this visit, the same procedure will take place, with the hand-held device scanning first your knee and then your neck. An IV may be placed in your wrist or arm and another radiotracer called Technitium-99m given. The radiology technician will use a special camera (called a gamma camera) that detects radioactive energy emitted from the thyroid gland and translates that into an image. The gamma camera will take multiple pictures from multiple angles, so remember to stay still when it's working. The image may have areas of hot and cold thyroid cells, or it may be completely normal. Some radiology departments also perform another image called a SPECT, or 3D imaging of the thyroid gland. The whole process will take thirty minutes to an hour.

AFTER THE SCAN

When the scan is complete, you may be asked to wait until the technologist checks the thyroid pictures in case additional images are needed. If you're told that additional images are needed, don't panic! The technologist is just trying to get the best pictures possible, and it doesn't necessarily mean that there was a problem. In fact, needing additional pictures is a common occurrence.

If you are breastfeeding, you should have already discussed a plan with the nuclear medicine team prior to the thyroid scan. With some radiotracers, you may be able to pump for seventy-two hours after the exam, storing the breast milk in the refrigerator for later use after allowing at least seventy-two hours of storage and radiotracer decay prior to giving the milk to your infant. Other radiotracers are not safe for infants, and the breastfeeding mother is encouraged to pump and dump for a time period after the scan.

After the scan, you can return to normal daily life without restrictions. You will usually hear results from your doctor in the days to weeks following the scan.

Allison's Experience: Thyroid Imaging

By the time I had a thyroid ultrasound, I had been experiencing pain and pressure in my throat and neck for several months. The results showed that I had two nodules and increased blood flow throughout my thyroid gland. This suggested inflammation or "thyroiditis," although I didn't yet have a diagnosis of AITD.

I had a second ultrasound done at Dr. Henderson's office, and because of her trained eye, she thought I was dealing with Hashimoto's, which a biopsy and an extremely high TPO antibody test confirmed. Because of my symptoms and increased thyroid blood flow, she also sent me for a thyroid uptake scan, which was quite high. Based on all the information, including negative testing for TRABs, Dr. Henderson realized that my high uptake number was *not* indicative of Graves', as some might think, but rather of a form of Hashimoto's: Hashitoxicosis. As stated in Chapter 3, this is one of the six major variants of Hashimoto's disease. Hashitoxicosis patients experience symptoms that usually vacillate between *hyper*thyroidism and *hypo*thyroidism.

I've continued to have ultrasound testing along the way. It's been a way to keep a check on what my thyroid is doing at any given time. Ultrasound testing is an effective method for visualizing, in concrete terms, the size and characteristics of nodules, the size of my thyroid itself, and ongoing inflammatory activity. I've had ultrasounds before treatment, during, and since, and although I don't need them as often now, we still look at my gland annually to make sure no new nodules have grown.

OTHER SCANS

There are several other less common scans that may be ordered in patients with AITD. These include: a CT scan, an MRI, or, uncommonly, a PET scan. Because these tests are infrequently ordered in AITD, we will not go into detail, but there are several things you should be aware of. Many times, abnormalities in the thyroid gland are found by accident after a CT scan or MRI is done for another reason, like for neck pain. If an abnormality is found, it is important to discuss next steps with your doctor. Sometimes CT scan and MRIs are ordered if you have a large goiter.

In some patients, the thyroid gland gets so large that it grows underneath the breastbone and wraps around the heart and airway. In these cases, your doctor may order a CT scan or MRI to determine how far down into the chest the thyroid goes. Less commonly, the thyroid gland may light up on a PET scan, which is typically performed in people who have had cancer. Hashimoto's glands can sometimes light up on PET scan because of chronic inflammation. Other times, there is a nodule in the thyroid that needs closer evaluation by a doctor. If you have thyroid findings on PET, it is important to work with your thyroid doctor to determine the next steps.

CONCLUSION

Imaging tests are some of the best diagnostic and monitoring tools for any-one who suspects they have AITD, or has been diagnosed with it. These tests are not painful, noninvasive, and are useful in providing considerable information. Many AITD patients have been through one or more type of imaging tests, as you may have been, if there are indicators that imaging would be useful. If you have imaging results that reveal an area of concern, your doctor may advise you to have a thyroid biopsy. We will learn more about this in the next chapter.

7.

Fine Needle Aspiration Biopsy and Molecular Testing

Up to this point, we have covered everything from exploring the history of thyroid disease to thyroid testing and diagnosis. We know that it is not uncommon for AITD patients to discover that they have a thyroid nodule. As previously stated, a great majority—over 95 percent—of thyroid nodules are completely benign, that is, non-cancerous. Many thyroid nodules or cysts look benign by thyroid ultrasound, and can be safely followed by an experienced thyroid doctor. Other nodules are too small to undergo thyroid biopsy and should also be followed with time to make sure that they do not grow. Still, others meet criteria to undergo fine needle aspiration (FNA) biopsy.

If your doctor recommends a fine needle aspiration biopsy—do not panic! We have written this chapter with you in mind and will walk you through the process so that you feel confident (and calm) when you arrive for your procedure. We will explore possible FNA results and the role of molecular testing in thyroid biopsy. At the conclusion of the chapter, you should feel confident in knowing what to expect with regards to the procedure and possible outcomes.

FINE NEEDLE ASPIRATION BIOPSY

Fine needle aspiration biopsy consists of a fine needle, smaller than what is used to draw blood, used to aspirate, or extract, thyroid cells. The needle is inserted through the skin of the neck and advanced just below the skin into the thyroid gland. The procedure is usually done in a medical office by a thyroid doctor, but can also be done in a radiology suite. FNA is recommended when thyroid ultrasound detects a thyroid nodule with one of the following characteristics:

- Large size (most nodules are over 1 cm)

- Increased blood flow (also referred to as vascular)

- Suspicious characteristics (See Chapter 6)

By performing an FNA procedure, your doctor can better determine whether your nodule is benign or cancerous and decide on next steps. So what does an FNA biopsy entail?

Before the Procedure

All medical practices are different, so make sure that you follow the specific instructions given to you by the doctor performing the procedure. Most often, there is no need to fast before the procedure, although you should eat something light so that you don't get nauseated. Additionally, you should take all prescribed medications and vitamins as you would normally.

As with the thyroid ultrasound discussed in Chapter 6, be sure to dress appropriately for the exam. Wear something lightweight, preferably a V-neck shirt or scoop neckline. You may be expected to change into a hospital gown. Do not wear a necklace or long, dangling earrings. Avoid the use of heavy foundation or concealer to the neck and the application of excessive perfume or cologne to the neck. If you have a very long beard, trim hair around the neck, or bring a hair tie to be able to move the beard out of the way before the exam.

Be sure to tell your doctor if you are allergic to any medications or to latex. Also, make sure you discuss whether you are on blood thinning medications like aspirin, Coumadin, Plavix, Heparin, Lovenox, or Eliquis. Sometimes, blood thinners may be stopped prior to the procedure, while many can be safely continued.

During The Procedure

During an FNA, it is usually expected that you will be able to lie flat with your neck extended for twenty to thirty minutes. If you have neck problems or are unable to lie flat, tell your doctor before the procedure. Sometimes, the FNA can be performed while sitting up. Once you are properly positioned, the procedure will begin.

STEP 1: *Cleaning Your Neck*

Someone will clean your neck with soap, alcohol, or cleaning solution to ensure that you don't get an infection. This process takes a couple of seconds and doesn't hurt.

STEP 2: *Numbing Your Neck*

Most of the time, your doctor will use numbing medication before proceeding with the FNA to reduce discomfort. Some physicians don't use numbing medication, believing that the numbing shot can be more uncomfortable than the actual procedure. If you would like to have numbing, ask for this before the procedure begins. Numbing is usually achieved with topical cream, cold spray, or a numbing shot, similar to what is given prior to a dental procedure. After about thirty seconds, the skin will feel numb to touch, which will make the FNA more comfortable.

STEP 3: *Swallowing*

Every time you swallow, the thyroid moves up and down in the neck. To ensure that the doctor can accurately target the thyroid nodule without it moving, purposely swallow before the needle is inserted. After the needle is in the thyroid, try your best not to swallow, to talk, breath heavily, or move. If you accidentally cough or swallow, don't panic. Just be aware that staying still during the procedure will help ensure the biopsy is performed properly.

STEP 4: *The "Needle" Part*

Now that you are numb, the needle prick should not be painful or sharp. You will still feel some pressure as the needle is inserted. The needle will be in the thyroid nodule for a couple of seconds, and during this time, you may feel the doctor move it in a rhythmic up-and-down motion. This up-and-down motion allows the thyroid cells to easily break free from the thyroid nodule so that they can be drawn in, removed, and examined. Besides feeling some pressure, there should be no pain. If you have pain, ask your doctor for more numbing medicine. You may feel some strange sensations in your jaw or ear—this is normal. These sensations will go away rather quickly after the needle is removed.

STEP 5: *Collecting Your Cells*

Doctors usually need to do several needle insertions (we call these "passes") into different parts of the thyroid nodule. The exact number of passes depends on how big the nodule is and how easily the doctor is able to collect the cells. Performing multiple passes ensures that enough material is collected for diagnosis and allows cells to be sampled from different parts of the nodule. In between passes, you can swallow and talk as you normally would. Just remember to swallow before the next pass is performed. During the procedure, remember to take slow, shallow breaths and only hold your breath if you are instructed to do so. The whole entire process should take no more than five to ten minutes.

STEP 6: *Checking Your Cells*

Many thyroid doctors and radiologists now have the ability to immediately check the cells under a microscope. This is important because it allows the doctor to know if he or she got enough cells for the pathologist to give you a diagnosis. If there are not enough cells, the performing physician may need to do several additional passes. If there are enough cells, the procedure is complete, and the tissue samples will then be sent to a pathology lab for interpretation. The results will be given to your doctor, who will then contact you.

After the Procedure

After the FNA procedure, you will be allowed to sit up and relax. You may be instructed to avoid taking aspirin or other blood thinners for a specified amount of time. Always ask your doctor. If you experience tenderness, use over-the-counter pain relievers—with your doctor's approval—and apply heat/cold to the area. It is normal to sometimes experience a small amount of swelling or bruising. All of these symptoms should resolve within forty-eight to seventy-two hours. Monitor for rash, fever, or severe swelling at the site and, if these occur, seek medical attention. Once the procedure is complete, you will likely be discharged home.

FNA Results

So what are the possible test results you can receive from a thyroid FNA? Because we are only collecting a small amount of thyroid cells (sometimes as few as sixty cells, and your body is made of trillions!), we can't know with 100-percent certainty if the thyroid nodule is benign or cancerous.

Allison's Experience: Thyroid Biopsy— Not as Bad as You Think

I knew that because I had thyroid nodules and symptoms, there was a chance I would need a thyroid biopsy. So I wasn't surprised when Dr. Henderson told me she'd recommend FNA—but I *was* nervous. The idea of anyone sticking a needle into my neck and pulling out samples of my thyroid was nerve-wracking, but not nearly as stress-inducing as not knowing if I had thyroid cancer or not.

Dr. Henderson applied numbing spray to my neck. "Spray a little extra," I joked. She used a hollow needle to extract samples from my thyroid nodule several times. "You're doing great," she said. "Almost done." Even as she was focused on the task at hand, she was reassuring. It wasn't pleasant, but it wasn't horrible either. It was uncomfortable, with a feeling of pressure, but not pain.

When she had adequate samples, she looked at them microscopically and told me that she could see that I had Hashimoto's, just as she had suspected. But she still had to send it to pathology to get the definitive report, to make sure there wasn't cancer involved. Two days later, my cell phone rang. It was Dr. Henderson. She called to tell me there was no cancer, but it definitely was Hashimoto's, and I would need to come back to discuss a plan going forward.

If I had let me fear of the biopsy dissuade me from having it done, I wouldn't have as much as information as possible about my condition—or all the facts needed for the best treatment plan to be developed.

While cancer is most often detected through FNA, there are times it can be missed (zero to 4 percent of the time), due to the small amount of cells removed. An FNA might show non-cancerous cells from the particular area that was biopsied, while a different part of the nodule could still be cancerous. Therefore, the only way to know with certainty a nodule is cancerous, is when a thyroid is surgically removed and the nodule and surrounding thyroid tissue is microscopically examined. Because thyroid nodules are so common and usually benign, we elect to perform FNA biopsies of different parts of the thyroid nodule instead of surgery to give us clues as to the nature of the nodule. Of course, you don't want to lose any part of your thyroid gland unless you have to.

In order to classify FNA results easily, we have broken down the possible results into six categories called the Bethesda categories—each with an associated risk of thyroid cancer. The lower the risk, the more confident doctors are that the nodule is benign; the higher the risk, the higher the likelihood of thyroid cancer. Once you know what the categories are and their associated risk of cancer, we will dive deeper into each category and possible next steps.

TABLE 7.1. THE BETHESDA CATEGORIES AND ASSOCIATED RISK	
BETHESDA CATEGORY	RISK OF CANCER
Category 1: Insufficient	It may need to be repeated
Category 2: Benign	Very Low (0 to 4 percent)
Category 3: Indeterminate, AUS/FLUS*	Low (5 to 15 percent)
Category 4: Indeterminate, Follicular Neoplasm	Moderate (15 to 30 percent)
Category 5: Suspicious for Cancer	High (60 to 75 percent)
Category 6: Cancer	Almost Certain (97 to 99 percent)

* AUS: Atypia of Undetermined Significance. FLUS: Follicular Lesion of Undetermined Significance.
Table adapted from The Bethesda System for Reporting Thyroid Cytopathology, 2009.

If you have already had an FNA, your doctor probably called you with one of the results in Table 7.1. Without a background on what the different diagnoses mean, it may have been difficult to grasp what exactly was found on your FNA biopsy. Here we will review each Bethesda category, interpretation, and discuss possible next steps.

CATEGORY 1: *Insufficient FNA*

This category can be frustrating to patients. The result really depends on what the nodule looks like by ultrasound. An insufficient FNA result can either be good, indicating benignity, or can mean that not enough cells were collected and that the FNA procedure needs to be repeated. For example, if a biopsy is performed on a simple thyroid cyst full of fluid, you will most likely get this result because the thyroid nodule is full of fluid, not cells. In this instance, the FNA is not typically repeated. If this result is obtained for a more solid nodule, it is more likely that the FNA will need to be repeated.

Sometimes nodules that are heavily calcified can have insufficient results, because cells are difficult to aspirate from them. If you get an FNA result that is insufficient, discuss next steps with your treating doctor.

CATEGORY 2: *Benign FNA*

This is the result we are hoping for when we do the biopsy. Thankfully, an overwhelming majority of biopsies come back in this category. Even with a benign FNA, it is important to follow the thyroid nodule by serial ultrasound over time to ensure that it doesn't grow or change. Although a benign result is reassuring, up to four patients in one hundred with a benign result will actually have thyroid cancer that was not picked up at initial biopsy.

Therefore, the American Thyroid Association recommends that these nodules be followed by ultrasound every couple of years. If the nodule grows, a repeat FNA is often recommended. Nodule growth doesn't necessarily imply malignancy; even benign nodules grow with time. On the other hand, if the nodule remains stable in size and appearance, both patient and physician are reassured that the lesion is, indeed, benign.

CATEGORIES 3 AND 4: *Indeterminate FNA*

So what does an "indeterminate" result actually mean? Indeterminate means that most of the cells from your nodule look normal, but there may be some unusual features. For example, the cells may be larger than expected. In other cases, there may be an absence of something called colloid (a normal finding on biopsy) or too many cells for the pathologist to feel comfortable calling the nodule benign. Just remember, if you get an indeterminate biopsy, you still have a 70- to 95-percent chance that the nodule is benign.

There are two indeterminate categories: Bethesda 3 and Bethesda 4. The categories are divided to more accurately predict likelihood of malignancy, with Bethesda 3 being more likely benign than Bethesda 4. In both instances, further testing is needed. In the past, almost all patients with indeterminate biopsies underwent surgical removal. Today, a majority of FNA samples in this category are first sent for molecular testing to determine whether surgery is necessary. We will discuss molecular testing in further detail later in the chapter.

A word of caution: If your results are inconclusive and a diagnosis can't be quickly made, but you have a noticeable lump that is growing at a rapid pace, you must be your own advocate and seek out another opinion *as soon as possible*. Although most of the time thyroid cancer is slow-growing, there are rare types of thyroid cancer that can enlarge rapidly, and surgical treatment is needed quickly.

CATEGORIES 5 AND 6: *Suspicious for Malignancy and Malignant*

A Category 5 or 6 nodule is cancer until proven otherwise. Therefore, a good majority of patients in this category undergo surgical excision. If you have a Bethesda 5 or 6 nodule, it is important to discuss with your doctor whether any additional imaging, usually an ultrasound or CT scan, is needed prior to surgery. In many cases, a thorough neck ultrasound through a procedure known as *lymph node mapping* can detect whether there are abnormal lymph nodes that also need to be removed at surgery. Lymph node mapping is important because, if a thyroid nodule is cancerous, it tends to spread first to surrounding neck lymph nodes. Removing all cancerous nodules and lymph nodes at the initial surgery is best.

Nobody wants to hear that they possibly have cancer. If you do have a Bethesda 5 or 6 result, however, it is important to know that most thyroid cancers grow extremely slowly over months to years. Therefore, in most cases it is safe to schedule surgery in the weeks to months following diagnosis, though you should discuss this with your treating physician.

Most thyroid cancers are so slow-growing, in fact, that some doctors recommend that small, nonaggressive thyroid cancers be closely monitored by ultrasound instead of undergoing immediate surgical removal. Less commonly, thyroid cancer may be more aggressive and need expedited removal. Be sure to discuss next steps with your treating physician. Most thyroid cancers are cured with surgical removal, but we will discuss other treatments, like radioactive iodine therapy and alcohol ablation, in further detail in Chapter 13.

Molecular Testing in Thyroid Disease

Remember our discussion on your genes? Science has made many advances in molecular medicine, meaning the study of how your genes contribute to development of disease. For patients with indeterminate thyroid nodules, an increasing number of medical centers are now using gene testing to determine whether the nodule is cancerous or benign. The genes that we test for are not the genes inherited from your mother and father; instead, we test for gene changes that can occur within the thyroid that lead to development of thyroid cancer.

There are multiple commercially available molecular tests that can be performed on indeterminate nodules. When negative for gene mutations or alterations, the nodules can be safely followed by ultrasound for growth. When positive, molecular testing can help to determine whether continued ultrasound surveillance is appropriate or whether the nodule should be surgically removed. If you have a Bethesda 3 or 4 nodule, you may wish to discuss molecular testing with your doctor.

CONCLUSION

It is not uncommon to have an FNA if you have thyroid nodules that are large, vascular, or suspicious. Remember, just because your doctor recommends having this procedure, doesn't mean that you have thyroid cancer. And although having an invasive procedure isn't welcome by anyone, it's very useful for the diagnosis related to thyroid nodules. FNA is relatively quick, usually without any complications, and typically provides invaluable information. For those patients whose results are indeterminate, where biopsy alone is not conclusive, the advanced technology of molecular testing can be used to further determine whether nodules are benign or cancerous. The clarity provided by both FNA and molecular testing can help patients to avoid unnecessary surgery and optimize thyroid care.

PART 3

Treatment
and Management

8.

Thyroid Replacement Medication

If you or a loved one has AITD, you may already have spent some time researching different formulations of thyroid hormone replacement medicine. Alternatively, you may have been prescribed a specific thyroid medicine without even realizing that there were many options to choose from.

In this chapter, we will explore all the available thyroid replacement options, explain the differences, and discuss how to find the medication that may be best suited for you. As we move through the material in this chapter, remember that every patient is different. There is no one-size-fits-all approach to thyroid replacement medication and dosing.

MANY THYROID REPLACEMENT OPTIONS

Did you know that Synthroid, a medication used for hypothyroidism, is the most commonly prescribed medicine in the United States? At 21.5 million prescriptions per month, it has remained at the top spot for years. This number is staggering and reflects the vast number of people in our country affected by thyroid disease. Unbelievably, this incredibly high number doesn't even account for patients taking different formulations of thyroid hormones. Here we will explore the different forms of thyroid replacement medicine, presenting pros and cons of each, in an effort to bring you one step closer to finding the thyroid medication that is right for you.

T4 Formulations

Similar to the way the thyroid gland produces hormones, thyroid replacement medicine is broken down into both T4 and T3 formulations. Remember, in the normal thyroid gland, 80 percent of thyroid hormone released into circulation is T4, or inactive thyroid hormone, and is converted by the body (with the help of DIO) to T3, or active hormone. Many physicians will start with T4-only formulations, assuming that your body will be able to convert the medicine appropriately to T3. While many healthy people are able to do this just fine, others have circumstances (medical conditions, vitamin deficiencies, interfering medications, and genetic changes) that make it hard for them to effectively use T4-only medications. In these cases, patients may need to add T3 or start a combination T4/T3 medication (more on this later in the chapter). Assuming that you have no other health concerns or contributing factors, T4-only medication is a good place to start.

Levothyroxine

Levothyroxine is the most commonly prescribed T4-only medication. On average, patients pay as little as $3.00 per month, though out-of-pocket cost can be as high as $20. With levothyroxine, it is important to know that there are many manufacturers and formulations that are re-packaged by different corporations. Why is this important? Because different manufacturers can have slightly different amounts of T4 per pill and can have different additives that can change how you absorb the medicine (more of this later in the chapter).

If you are prescribed levothyroxine, it is helpful to ask your pharmacist which manufacturer he or she uses, so you can be well informed about what you are taking. If your pills start to look different (different shape or initials on the medicine) or the pharmacist notifies you of a switch in the manufacturer, it is important to tell your doctor so that your thyroid labs can be checked to ensure that the new pill has not affected your thyroid levels.

Most T4 formulations use dyes in their medicine to help patients identify the different dosages. For example, the 100 mcg tablet is yellow, whereas the 200 mcg tablet is pink. If you are sensitive to dyes, or don't wish to be exposed to dyes daily, then you may wish to ask about the 50 mcg tablet that is white and does not contain added dyes. If you have difficulty swallowing pills, most T4 formulations, with the exception of the brand Tirosint, can be crushed and dissolved in water for easy administration.

Synthroid

Synthroid is the most commonly prescribed brand formulation of generic levothyroxine. Studies have demonstrated that there may be slight differences in how Synthroid is absorbed compared to generic forms of levothyroxine. The Food & Drug Administration (FDA) considers thyroid medicine to have narrow therapeutic index, meaning the level at which it is effective is very close to the level where it can have toxic effects. Therefore, it's important that levothyroxine generics are extremely close to name brand formulations.

Even though these medicines are similar in dosing, all of them (name brand and generic alike) are absorbed by the body slightly differently. Some generic levothyroxine formulations are slightly stronger (at the same dosage) than Synthroid, and vice versa. Therefore, if you are switched from generic to name brand or name brand to generic, it is important to check your thyroid levels to ensure that you are getting the correct dose.

The American Thyroid Association (ATA), American Association for Clinical Endocrinologists (AACE), and the Endocrine Society issued a warning statement to providers and patients when Synthroid was made generic in 2004, stressing the importance of sticking to the same formulation, as even slight alterations of medicine can significantly affect thyroid levels.

Thyroid Quick Tip: You can take generic levothyroxine or name brand Synthroid as long as you take your dose as prescribed and limit changes in manufacturers. If you don't want to have to deal with changes in generic manufacturers (and potential impact on your thyroid function), stick with the name brand.

Levoxyl

Levoxyl is a different name brand T4-only medication, similar to name brand Synthroid. It is packaged slightly differently with different types of binders, thereby slightly affecting absorption. Some patients do better with Levoxyl than they do with generic levothyroxine or Synthroid. Reasons are likely due to a gentler rate of absorption, better tolerance of fillers, or the fact that Levoxyl is gluten- and lactose-free.

Tirosint

Tirosint is a name brand T4-only medication that is unique in the fact that it is a gel capsule instead of a tablet. This is good for two reasons. One, it can help with faster absorption in the gut if there is an absorption issue. Two, it has fewer fillers that any of the other T4-only formulations (including no dyes!). The downside? It is currently much more expensive than some of the other formulations. Still, for those with commercial insurance, most drug companies have patient co-pay cards that you can find online that help reduce the monthly cost.

Other T4 Formulations

Other forms of T4-only medications include Unithroid, Levo-T, and compounded T4. All of the T4-only formulations use synthetic T4, with slightly different packaging. The Food & Drug Administration (FDA) approves all commercially available T4 medication, with the exception of compounded T4. If you are prescribed a T4-only medicine, you should work with your doctor to make sure that you are on the best formulation for your body and that your thyroid levels are optimized. We will discuss thyroid hormone optimization further in Chapter 12.

T3-Only Formulations

In Chapter 5, we discussed how some medications and diseases interfere with T4 to T3 conversion. Therefore, patients with interfering medications or diseases may not do as well with T4-only medications. Typically, these patients continue with hypothyroid symptoms (despite normal TSH levels), along with low or low-normal serum T3 levels. In many instances, these patients do better with addition of T3 to their T4-only medications or with T4/T3 combination therapies. Here we will discuss available thyroid hormone options for patients who also require T3.

Cytomel

Cytomel is the most commonly available form of name brand T3. It is short acting and is best dosed twice a day. Because it is short acting, some patients will get T3 symptoms a couple of hours after taking it. Cytomel is not gluten-free. Typically, Cytomel is added to T4-only medication in a 4:1 ratio, increasing T3 levels and improving patient symptoms.

Liothyronine

Liothyronine is the generic formulation of T3. It is gluten-free and has less allergy inducing fillers than name brand Cytomel. It works similarly and is dosed in a 4:1 fashion, along with T4-only medicine. Very rarely, patients are placed on T3-only medication without T4, but this is usually just for a short time prior to thyroid cancer treatment. Otherwise, it is most commonly used in combination with T4 in an effort to replenish both T4 and T3 stores.

Other Forms of T3-Only Medicines

Sometimes, patients can't tolerate the fillers or get T3 symptoms with the commercially available T3 formulations. In these cases, individualized T3 formulations with immediate- or sustained-release action can help replenish T3 stores while decreasing side effects. These formulations are called "compounds" and are created at compounding pharmacies. The downside? These custom blended medications are more expensive, take longer time to make, and are more prone to dosing errors.

If you and your doctor decide on compounded medication, make sure that you're working with a Pharmacy Compounding Accreditation Board (PCAB) pharmacy that uses a PCCA starting material (just call the pharmacy and ask). Sometimes, these PCCA starters can be placed on backorder or are hard to find, so make sure that your pharmacy notifies you if there is a change in how they make your medicine (similar to how you should be aware of the T4 generic manufacturers).

T4/T3 Combination Therapies

In addition to adding T3 to T4 only therapy, T4/T3 combination therapies are also available and are widely popular among those interested in more natural approaches. Most available formulations are derived from pig or cow thyroid glands and contain T4 and T3 together in one pill. Here we discuss available thyroid hormone options for patients on combination treatment.

Armour

Armour Thyroid is the most common type of T4/T3 combination treatment. Armour Thyroid is a brand name formulation of desiccated pig thyroid gland. "Desiccated" means that the pig's thyroid gland is removed, mashed up, and placed into a pill formulation. Because it is animal-derived, it is thought to be a more natural approach to thyroid replacement. It is still, however, made in a laboratory where fillers are added to the medicine to put it into pill form. Armour is currently not FDA-approved (we will discuss this later in the chapter), but it is regulated in regard to how many micrograms of T4 and T3 are in every pill.

Thyroglobulin and thyroid peroxidase (TPO) proteins, as well as other thyroid metabolites, are detectable in the Armour formulation. Most of these additional metabolites are inactive and don't have a significant effect on the body, although some reports suggest there may be a theoretical increase in TPOAbs and TgAbs in AITD patients taking these medicines. Some patients do excellent on the Armour Thyroid formulation, with complete resolution of their hypothyroid symptoms. Other patients can't tolerate the foul taste or have significant T3 symptoms. (See Chapter 5.)

For all desiccated pig thyroid formulations, it is important to remember that the pig ratio T4 to T3 ratio is 1:1. This is significantly different than the human T4 to T3 ratio of 4:1. Because of this difference, it is common to see patients on desiccated thyroid hormone who have very high T3 levels but very low T4 levels (for example, they have a lot of cash in their wallet, but not a lot of reserve in their thyroid bank). Therefore, some patients are placed on levothyroxine in addition to Armour Thyroid to help with their T4 stores. Regardless, every patient is different; some feel their best on Armour Thyroid, while others feel better with an alternate form of thyroid medication. In all circumstances, it is imperative that patients work with their doctor to find the formulation that is right for them. For those patients who keep Kosher or Halal, using material sourced from pigs may present an issue.

Nature-Throid

Nature-Throid— and yes, it is spelled this way—is a similar T4/T3 combination medication that also uses desiccated pig but is packaged differently than Armour. Some patients tolerate this formulation better than Armour Thyroid, likely because different binders and fillers affect how different people absorb the medication. There is a trace amount of lactose present in Nature-Throid, though likely at too small a concentration to really cause issues in those who are lactose-intolerant.

Regardless, patients should be aware of any new changes in how they're feeling when taking any of the thyroid replacement options, as it may indicate a medicine intolerance (symptoms may include bloating, diarrhea, constipation, or headache, and usually occur hours after ingestion). The T4:T3 ratio and dosing in Nature-Throid is the same as Armour Thyroid, although most patients report feeling differently when they switch between formulations. Again, this is likely due to differences in fillers and individual patient differences in medication absorption (due to differences in gut absorption and the gut microbiome—more on this in Chapter 9).

NP Thyroid

NP Thyroid (Acella) is another form of desiccated thyroid hormone. This medicine is somewhat unique in the fact that it has fewer fillers and can be absorbed sublingually (under the tongue), which is helpful for people who have trouble swallowing pills. Also, it is more affordable than some other formulations.

Other T4/T3 Combination Formulations

Similar to levothyroxine generic, Thyroid USP is the generic type of T4/T3 desiccated thyroid medication. Dosing is similar to all of the name brand formulations, although fillers and individual rates of absorption may vary. Additional formulations include WP Thyroid, Westhroid, and compounded T4/T3, among others.

What Could Happen If I Miss Medication or Choose Not to Take Any?

Some patients are truly medication adverse, and have difficulty tolerating any of the previously mentioned medications. If you have subclinical hypothyroidism and minimal symptoms, you and your doctor may elect to follow your levels without using medications. He or she may also recommend dietary changes and vitamins (more about that in Chapters 9 and 10). However, if you are symptomatic, you may be advised to start thyroid medicine. Normalizing your thyroid levels will not only help improve your AITD symptoms, but taking thyroid medicine to optimize your TSH is the most effective way to lower your TPO and Tg antibodies, thereby improving the autoimmune attack on your thyroid gland. (More on this in Chapter 12.)

Patients with hypothyroidism often ask what would happen if they miss occasional doses or don't take the medicine at the same time each day. Know that it is important to always take your medicine as prescribed. Missing a couple of days should not dramatically affect your thyroid health and is not typically dangerous, but the medicine should be started back as soon as possible. Missing more than an occasional dose, however, can dramatically affect your levels. Always discuss missed doses with your doctor and keep him or her informed of any interruptions in thyroid dosing. Taking the medicine at the same time of day is important for T3-only and T4/T3 combination medicines; but less important for T4-only medicines. This is because T4 medicines are longer acting in the body.

Many patients also wonder what would happen if there were ever a national shortage of thyroid replacement medicine or an inability to get the medication. Hopefully this will never happen, but in the worst case scenario, ingesting animal thyroid gland is a proven effective option for thyroid dosing.

Patients can live without a thyroid gland, but not well. Longstanding, severe hypothyroidism (usually persistent over many years) can lead to *myxedema coma*, a condition of mental confusion, low body temperature, swelling, congestive heart failure, and severe, life-threatening organ failure. If you are prescribed thyroid medicine, it is extremely important to take the medicine, as you can get very sick if you fail to do so. Patients who have had only part of their thyroid removed, as opposed to the entire gland, may not get as sick as those without a thyroid gland, but can still develop severe hypothyroid symptoms if they don't take their medicine. Therefore, finding a thyroid replacement option with minimal side effects that leads to normal thyroid levels and overall well-being is of vital importance.

Why Do Some Doctors Stick to Synthroid?

This chapter raises the question, "If there are so many thyroid replacement options, why do all doctors seem to stick to Synthroid?" Conspiracy theories aside—and no, your doctor doesn't get a kickback for prescribing Synthroid—most physicians want to stick to professional guidelines and prescribe FDA-regulated medicine. They do this because they took the Hippocratic Oath when they became doctors, pledging to "first, do no harm."

Sometimes, this preoccupancy with guidelines and FDA regulation can cause delays in physicians adopting thyroid hormone replacement options that actually do work—sometimes better.

The point to remember is that thyroid hormone dosing is very technical and, if done incorrectly, particularly with the T3 and T4/T3 combination therapies, can cause dramatic, life-altering symptoms. Therefore, it is of utmost importance to seek out an experienced thyroid doctor who is well versed in thyroid hormone replacement options and optimization of thyroid levels. Note that while *compounded* T3, T4 and combination T3/T4 require a compounding pharmacy, all others are available at regular pharmacies.

FDA REGULATION

The Food & Drug Agency is an arm of the federal government. They explain their role as being "responsible for protecting the public health by ensuring the safety, efficacy, and security of human and veterinary drugs, biological products, and medical devices." But what does that actually mean?

When prescription and over-the-counter medications have FDA approval, it means that they have undergone a review process and been deemed to have benefits which outweigh the risks. It does *not* mean that the FDA has independently tested the medication. They don't do independent testing, but rather, rely on the materials, research, and testing of the drug manufacturer who submitted the approval request. FDA approval also doesn't mean that a drug is completely safe, as there are risks associated with every medication.

So, what does it mean if a drug is not FDA approved? The fact that a drug has not gained FDA approval does not mean it's a bad drug. It means that for a variety of possible reasons, the FDA has not found that it meets the criteria for approval. Furthermore, some unapproved drugs are allowed to be sold. However, these medications are typically not covered by insurance companies.

How does this affect you and other Hashimoto's patients? Let's go over the medications used by thyroid patients. This list reflects the current state of FDA approvals, but it is subject to change. For instance, Armour used to have FDA approval, but has since been removed from the list of FDA approved drugs.

Remember, FDA approval is not the only criteria you should consider when deciding what is best for your specific situation. Working closely with an open minded and informed doctor is the best way to address your specific thyroid medication needs.

TABLE 8.1. THYROID MEDICATIONS FDA APPROVED/NOT APPROVED			
FDA APPROVED		**NOT FDA APPROVED**	
Levothyroxine	Unithroid	Armour	Westhroid
Synthroid	Levo-T	Nature-Throid	WP Thyroid
Levoxyl	Liothyronine	NP Thyroid	Compounded Medicine
Tirosint	Cytomel	Thyroid USP	

A Thyroid Replacement Story

Remember Mrs. Jones? She was diagnosed with Hashimoto's back in Chapter 3. At first, she tried levothyroxine, the generic form of Synthroid, but still had daily symptoms. After several months, she was switched to Armour Thyroid. She feels great and is back to her normal, energetic self, whereas on levothyroxine she felt sluggish and weak. Today she is having lunch with her friend Mrs. Smith, who is also on levothyroxine and not feeling 100 percent. Because of her own experience, she advises Mrs. Smith to ask her doctor for Armour Thyroid. Her physician, wanting to help her achieve good thyroid health, agrees to switch her to Armour. After two weeks on the medication, Mrs. Smith has gone from feeling sluggish to having severe high T3 symptoms.

She describes heart palpitations and a tight feeling in her chest, as well as worsening anxiety. She has no issues with her adrenal axis (more on this later), nor does she have any other contributing medical conditions. She does not like her new T3 symptoms with Armour Thyroid and ends up switching back to levothyroxine. After coming off her Armour Thyroid and optimizing (for example, increasing) her levothyroxine dose, Mrs. Smith is back to normal and feels better than she has felt in years.

This type of scenario happens all the time in clinical thyroid practice. It is important to realize that some patients do better on T4 only, whereas others do better on T4/T3 combination therapy. Other patients do best on both T4 and T3 replacement, dosed separately. Patients like Mrs. Smith oftentimes don't need to switch medicines, but simply need to optimize their thyroid dosage to feel better. Other times, patients need to try multiple formulations before they find one that works with their body chemistry.

Thyroid Quick Tip: There is no one-size-fits-all approach to thyroid replacement medication. Everyone is different! It is important to work with your thyroid doctor in finding the formulation that is right for you.

FILLERS IN THYROID MEDICATION

In addition to differing amounts of active ingredients, each thyroid replacement option also has a list of different fillers that can cause side effects in sensitive individuals. Fillers are substances within the medication capsule that influence the stability of the thyroid medicine and can influence your body's absorption of the medication. The most commonly reported side effects from medication fillers include rash, bloating/diarrhea and headache. A list of common fillers that may cause human allergies or sensitivities are listed in Tables 8.2. and 8.3.

TABLE 8.2. COMMON T4 FORMULATIONS					
	GLUTEN	**LACTOSE**	**CORN**	**SUCROSE**	**DYES****
Levothyroxine	X*	X	X*	X*	X
Synthroid		X	X		X
Unithroid		X	X		X
Levoxyl					X
Compounded T4			X*		
Tirosint					

* Select manufacturers (for levothyroxine generic, Lannett and Mylan are gluten-free)
** All strengths except for the 50 mcg strength

TABLE 8.3. COMMON T4/T3 AND T3 ONLY FORMULATIONS					
	GLUTEN	**LACTOSE**	**CORN**	**SUCROSE**	**DYES**
Armour			X		
Nature-throid		X			
NP Thyroid					
WP Thyroid		X			
Compounded T3			X*		
Cytomel	X		X	X	
Liothyronine			X*		

* Select manufacturers (liothyronine manufactured by Sigma Pharma has corn)

Gluten is derived from modified food starch, which is used as filler. Lactose is typically found as lactose monohydrate and is usually present in minuscule amounts. Much of the corn is from microcrystalline cellulose or cellulose (although some cellulose is derived from non-corn products), but some medications have actual corn starch added.

Weighing the Options

As you can see, there are multiple things to consider prior to selecting a thyroid medication. In Table 8.4, we have constructed a table listing the pros and cons of each therapy option to help you in your decision-making process. There are no perfect formulations, but there are medicines that can help optimize your thyroid health.

Which Thyroid Medication Is Best?

We have presented a lot of information on the different types of thyroid medicine. You might be throwing your hands in the air saying, "Okay, but which one is best? Which one would you choose?" Remember, everyone is different! You may have a genetic make-up that needs extra T3 to feel back to normal, or you may be very sensitive to T3 absorption and need a T4-only formulation.

Contributing medications, supplements, and other medical conditions can dramatically impact thyroid hormone metabolism (refer to Chapter 5 for a review). Nutrient deficiencies, food intolerances, and gut health also impact tolerance of thyroid medicine (more on this in Chapter 9). The biggest take away is that there is no one-size-fits-all approach. All aspects of medicine today are moving towards a more personalized approach, which makes sense because you are uniquely you and your thyroid medication and dosing should be prescribed accordingly.

Finding the Right Formulation For You

Some patients do very well with the initial type of medicine they are prescribed. They don't need very many changes in dosing and always feel pretty good. Others have a harder time finding the optimal thyroid dose, particularly if there are changes in other contributing medical conditions or the addition of new medications. In any case, it is important

TABLE 8.4. PROS AND CONS OF T4-ONLY, T4 PLUS T3-ONLY, AND T4/T3-COMBINATION THERAPY		
T4-ONLY	**T4+T3 ONLY**	**T4/T3 COMBO**
PROS		
FDA approved	Can be dosed physiologically for being a human (4:1 ratio of T4:T3)	One pill
Cheapest		More natural
One pill		No dyes
Least side effects	Can increase T3 levels in poor T4 to T3 converters	Less fillers
CONS		
Relies on your body to convert to T3	Two pills	Expensive
	Fillers and dyes	Not FDA regulated
Not good in patients with poor T4 to T3 conversion	Needs an experienced doctor for dosing	More T3 symptoms and side effects
Fillers and dyes		Not 4:1 T4:T3 ratio

to work with an experienced thyroid doctor who is open-minded and works as a partner in your thyroid care. AITD is a lifelong condition (even those that go into remission—see Chapter 12—can have flares down the road). That's why finding a lifelong thyroid doctor that you trust is of utmost importance.

Thyroid Quick Tip: If you are sensitive to medications, have reactions to fillers, or have known food sensitivities, you may wish to take thyroid hormone formulations that have limited fillers or no fillers added.

Insurance Considerations

There are several insurance considerations to be aware of, as it relates to thyroid medications. If a drug is not FDA approved, or on the company's annual preferred medication list, it may not be covered by insurance. If your doctor requests name brand only for your prescription, your insurance may initially deny this request. In either scenario, you can ask your doctor if they would be willing to request authorization for the unapproved drug. If your doctor can explain why you have a legitimate need for a certain medication, the insurance company might approve it. Sometimes insurance companies will ask that you try their "preferred" thyroid medicines first, and fail them, before they will approve the request.

If the insurance company denies the request, you may end up paying out-of-pocket for the medicine. Compounded medications, in particular, are almost always paid for out-of-pocket. Some pharmaceutical companies offer patient assistance and discount cards for patients who have a financial need. Many brand name prescriptions will have patient discount cards available on their websites to help cut costs (to find these just Google the drug name). It's best to ask your doctor or pharmacist if they're aware of such assistance programs, or to contact the drug manufacturer to inquire directly.

The Future of Thyroid Hormone Replacement

Current thyroid replacement options are not perfect. In a perfect world, T4 options would have fewer fillers, T3 options would be longer acting, and T4/T3 combination treatments would supply the correct T4:T3 ratio to human patients. In the future, affordable, consistent, and individualized compounded T4/T3 formulations based on a patient's body weight and other factors would be optimal for dosing. Even further down the road is the potential for thyroid cell transplant (*we are a long way off*), where administration of live thyroid cells could help to optimize and regulate thyroid hormone production in the body. In the meantime, we will continue to optimize thyroid levels with the tools we currently have, as we look towards the future of medicine.

CONCLUSION

When choosing thyroid medication, remember that there is no universally successful approach. Patients must work with their doctors to determine what medicine is right for them. When reading online blogs and message boards, it is important to keep this in mind. As you search for your thyroid doctor, look for a physician who is open minded and easy to work with—so that together, you can find the best formulation for your body and optimize your thyroid health.

In the future, new treatments and interventions will strive to influence the autoimmune process before it destroys the thyroid gland completely.

This is where the future of thyroid medicine is going. Some autoimmune triggers are not easily modifiable (for example, an untreatable viral infection that triggers longstanding autoimmunity), whereas others are modifiable (such as, treatment of nutrient deficiencies, changes to diet, and treatment of underlying bacterial infection). These modifiable lifestyle interventions are where we are going next on our thyroid journey.

9.

Hashimoto's Disease and Your Diet

Have you ever heard the expression "You are what you eat"? For AITD patients, this statement is particularly true. Thyroid function and autoimmunity can improve dramatically with proper diet and nutrition. Just like all cells in the body, both thyroid and immune cells need certain nutrients to work properly. In Chapter 2, for example, we discussed iodine deficiency as a cause of endemic thyroid goiter and hypothyroidism. Similar research has shown that vitamin D deficiency is strongly linked to immune dysfunction and autoimmune disease. Although many of these vitamins can be supplemented, it is important to first optimize thyroid nutrition and reduce autoimmunity by changing your diet.

If you search for dietary recommendations for Hashimoto's disease on the Internet, you will most likely find loads of conflicting information. In this chapter, we will give you a clear and understandable review of the dietary recommendations important to Hashimoto's patients, as well as the evidence behind them. This should help you to design a dietary plan with your doctor based on the latest information. Similar to thyroid replacement medicine, everyone is different in regards to the dietary recommendations needed to optimize immune function. Individual differences depend on genetics, Hashimoto's triggers, coexisting illnesses or medications, and alterations in bacteria that reside in the intestinal tract, which we will refer to from here on as the *gut microbiome*.

Our aim in this chapter is to give you practical information to make an impact in your nutritional status and immune health without overwhelming you with data. Although there is research in nutrition and autoimmunity, there are not many prospective, randomized controlled trials, which are considered the best kind of studies. Many of our recommendations are based on the results gathered from smaller studies, but some of our advice is just common sense.

THE GUT AND AUTOIMMUNITY

If we are going to talk about nutrition, we must start with your gut. The gut is the gastrointestinal tract, which is comprised of the gall bladder, intestines (small and large), liver, esophagus, pancreas, and stomach. However, when we refer to the gut in autoimmunity, we are primarily referring to the stomach and intestines. The intestines play a major role in digestion, with the small intestine absorbing most nutrients for the body's use. But did you know that the gut is also involved in immunity? In fact, the gut houses more immune cells than any other part of our body, up to 80 percent of your body's T and B cell soldiers!

There is good reason for this. Throughout your life, the gut is continuously exposed to foreign food-derived material. Just think of all the chemicals you can't pronounce on your food labels. Be aware that bacteria, viruses, and fungi are in your food, and pesticides reside on the surface of your fruits and vegetables. Immune cells are present to try to regulate this exposure and keep everything functioning properly.

Think of the immune cells in your gut as soldiers standing behind a stone wall, where the stone wall represents the lining of your intestine. When any substance passes through the gut, T cell and B cell soldiers are there to check identification before allowing these substances to pass through the intestine walls. With a healthy functioning gut, this process assures that vital nutrients are absorbed into the bloodstream, while waste products and non-nutrients are disposed of and foreign invaders are eliminated.

Now imagine your gut as a training boot camp, the place where your T cell soldiers and B cell snipers learn to identify friend and foe through continuous identification checks. Some are recognized as friend and are allowed through, while others are identified as foe and attacked. As you will learn, the curriculum at boot camp can become dramatically altered in a gut environment that is overwhelmed by foes. This unfriendly environment is not conducive to learning, prompting T and B cell "soldiers-in-training" to enter continuous fight mode before they're properly trained and contributing to autoimmunity. With this all-hands-on-deck mentality, chaos ensues, and you have a much higher chance of getting sick.

When your gut microenvironment is continuously exposed to foes, it remains in a chronic state of inflammation, putting your immune cell soldiers in continuous fight-mode instead of training-mode. In this situation, known by some as *leaky gut*, the gut is on high alert, producing large amounts of a protein called zonulin. Think of zonulin as a gate-keeper that opens established gates in the gut wall, called tight junctions. When the gates are open, more harmful particles pass through the gates. Once through the gates, they are recognized by T and B immune cells, which travel through the bloodstream—and an immune response is triggered throughout the body.

"Leaky gut" describes what happens with increased opening of the tight junctions, but the term can sometimes be misleading to patients, with some misinterpreting it. No, it doesn't mean that the hot dog you ate yesterday has leaked through your gut and is now floating around in your blood. Actually, leaky gut means that there is chronic inflammation and a lot of action at the gates in the stone wall. Therefore, it may be more accurate to refer to this altered gut state of chronic immune activation as *gut en garde* or, as we like to call it, *fighting gut*. In fighting gut, the intestinal wall isn't just passively leaking. Instead, it is mounting a full-fledged immune attack response against food particles and foreign substances, such as abnormal gut bacteria, food proteins, artificial ingredients, and infections that it sees as a threat.

The good news? You can prevent fighting gut and optimize your boot camp environment by reducing the number of foes traveling through the intestinal walls, allowing time for your soldiers to become properly trained, and positively impacting AITD. One of the first lessons we should learn when trying to treat AITD is that any inflammation in the body can worsen thyroid antibodies and the downstream immune attack on the thyroid. Therefore, putting your fighting gut back into its natural, peaceful state is an important place to start. So what keeps the gut healthy?

THE MICROBIOME AND HUMAN DISEASE

Did you know that there are 100 trillion bacteria residing in your gut right now? That's three to six times the number of cells in the human body. Gross, you may think! Actually, humans have evolved to live in a mutually beneficial relationship with these gut bacteria, called your *gut microbiome*.

The scientific community is just starting to understand how important this relationship truly is.

The gut microbiome lines our gut and feeds on our nutrients in order to survive. It also helps protect us from foreign invaders, such as abnormal bacteria, viruses, fungi, or chemicals—the "bad guys" that may make us sick. Therefore, you can think of the microbiome as our first line of defense against the foe, protecting the outside of our wall. These "good guy" bacteria also signal to our immune soldiers that the coast is clear, allowing our T and B soldiers to spend time in their training exercises to properly mature and become healthy immune cells that don't make us sick.

Therefore, maintaining a healthy gut microbiome is of utmost importance as our first line of defense against autoimmune thyroid disease. How do we do this? By feeding our good guys healthy nutrients and avoiding unhealthy nutrients that allow the bad guys to take over, resulting in a chronic state of fighting gut. We can feed our healthy gut microbiome in two ways—through diet and through the use of vitamins, which we will address further in Chapters 9 and 10. Let's start by focusing on diet.

MAINTAINING A HEALTHY DIET TO PREVENT FIGHTING GUT

If you have a fighting gut, it will take time and effort to restore peace at the stone wall. Not only do you have to remove the offending foes, but you have to restore adequate nutrition, quiet the inflammation, and correctly retrain your poor, exhausted soldiers. This can be done, but it takes time and persistence. We'll take you through the pertinent factors that influence gut health.

Food as Medicine in AITD

With all the diets circulating in the media and on the internet, it's no wonder that most patients are confused as to what they should be eating to maintain a healthy barrier and prevent or improve autoimmunity. That's why it's so important to feed your gut the correct food for healthy immune regulation.

Because we know everyone reacts differently to diet, based on an individual's genetics, microbiome, and immune system, there is no one-size-fits-all approach. There are, however, some foods that a majority of health experts agree are not optimal for human health. Not surprisingly, these same foods are also not optimal for thyroid health. Therefore, let's start with which foods to avoid.

Foods to Avoid in Hashimoto's

There is one simple rule for selecting foods if you have Hashimoto's:

Avoid foods that promote a state of gut inflammation or negatively impact thyroid hormone production, thereby contributing to or worsening AITD.

Many of the foods within this group are man-made, meaning that they automatically look foreign to our good guy bacteria and our immune soldiers. And as we said in the previous sections, these foreign proteins can act as foes that promote a state of chronic fighting gut, thereby promoting autoimmunity and AITD. Therefore, it stands to reason that, before making any other dietary recommendations, one must avoid foods that are perceived as foreign to the gut.

It is important to understand that processed foods, artificial sweeteners, and pesticides can all interfere with thyroid gland function by restricting iodine uptake or by acting as triggers to your immune system. The following products are detrimental to your health and should be avoided whenever possible. Let's discuss the food related "foes" that you need to know.

■ Foe #1: Processed Foods

Any food that is canned, dehydrated, or has chemicals added to it to enhance flavor, extend shelf life, or improve appearance is a processed food. In fact, up to sixty percent of the American diet is comprised of processed foods. It's easy to dismiss them as simply bagged chips, candy, or junk food. Instead, the list includes lunchmeat, sausage, bacon, margarines, dressings, peanut butter, dairy products, and almost everything on grocery shelves that comes in premade packaging.

Did you know that some of the ingredients in your processed food have been long associated with human disease, including the development of obesity, autoimmunity, and cancer? These man-made chemicals may make your foods look fresh, taste good, and last longer, but deep within the trenches of the gut your T and B cell soldiers are going to war. Table 9.1 shows some of the top offenders, and food items in which they are commonly found.

TABLE 9.1 INGREDIENTS TO STAY AWAY FROM		
INGREDIENT	**WHAT IT DOES**	**WHAT IT'S IN**
Artificial colors (Blue, Green, Red, Yellow, Caramel)	To change or enhance the color of food, making it more appealing. **Note:** *Read all labels for the words "blue, green, red, yellow, dye, or caramel coloring," and avoid foods which contain them.*	Canned soups, colored cereals, colored oatmeal, colored yogurt, salad dressings, farmed salmon (injected with dyes to make it pink), gelatin, pre-packaged popcorns, and sports drinks.
Butylated hydroxyanisole (BHA) and butylated hydroxytoluene (BHT)	Preservative used to keep fats and oils from becoming rancid. The Department of Health and Human Services refers to them as "reasonably anticipated to be a human carcinogen."	Baked goods, beer, butter, cereal, chewing gum, granola bars, instant mashed potatoes, lard, preserved meat, and potato chips.
High fructose corn syrup (HFCS)	HFCS is an artificial sweeter. It's a cheap substitute for white refined sugar, and is a staple of the American diet. It's in almost every sector of food.	Candy, cereal, condiments, frozen snack foods, granola bars, ice cream, store bought baked goods, TV dinners, and more.
Monosodium glutamate (MSG)	A flavor enhancer used to intensify the savory flavor of certain foods. **Note:** *Read all labels for words like "monosodium glutamate, hydrolyzed protein, autolyzed yeast, glutamic acid, and yeast extract."*	Beef jerky, Chinese food, chicken and beef flavoring, dressings and gravies, fast food, fried foods, low fat milk, potato chips, and salted flavored snacks.
Partially hydrogenated oils	These are added to increase shelf life and decrease need for refrigeration. These foods contain trans fat, which negatively affects cholesterol.	Baked goods, creamy peanut butter, coffee creamers, fried foods, margarine, packaged snack foods, pre-made dough, and vegetable shortening.
Sodium benzoate and potassium benzoate	Preservatives used to increase flavor, as well as extend shelf life, by inhibiting growth of yeast and mold. When combined with ascorbic acid (found in some sodas), these preservatives can form benzene, a known carcinogen.	Condiments, diet soda, fruit juice, jam, pickles, and salad dressing.
Sodium nitrates and sodium nitrites	These are added to extend shelf life and add color to food. Nitrates are generally not harmful, but there is a possible issue when the bacteria in our mouth and gut turns them into nitrites. Through a chemical process, those nitrites can then form nitrosamines, which are potentially harmful substances. Although further study is needed, it is believed that frequent consumption can be a contributing factor to cancer.	Bacon, hot dogs, beef jerky, and most lunch meat.

You are not alone if you're overwhelmed by this list. These ingredients are in a majority of the foods we eat. But with awareness and vigilance, it's possible to limit your exposure to these chemical food additives.

OUR ADVICE: Do your best and follow these three simple steps when trying to eliminate these artificial chemicals from your food:

Step 1. Home cooking. Making items by scratch allows you to use fresh ingredients and avoid artificial preservatives. If home cooking isn't an option for you, there are an increasing number of businesses that provide home delivery of fresh, organic meals.

Step 2. Focus on fresh. Spend most of your time in the fresh produce aisle of the grocery store or, even better, the local farmer's market.

Step 3. Look for labels with only a few ingredients. If you choose prepackaged foods, buy the item with the names of foods you actually recognize and the least number of ingredients on the label.

■ Foe #2: Sugar and Artificial Sweeteners

Sugar is linked to diabetes, obesity, heart disease, and inflammation. Foods with added sugar are worse than foods that contain their own natural sugar. And why is that? Sugar is a normal ingredient found in fruits and certain vegetables, but because there's also fiber in those foods, it takes longer for the sugar to be absorbed. Unfortunately, many people believe they are being healthier by using artificial sweeteners in place of sugar.

It is estimated that there are over a hundred different terms used on labels that are either sugar with a different name or artificial forms of sweetener. The sweeteners listed on the next page are all derived from different sources and created by using various processing methods. The majority of them are not normally sold to the general public, but rather are used as ingredients added into various food and drink products to provide sweetness.

All of the listed substances give food its sweet taste and may contribute to the worsening of your condition by promoting inflammation. Stevia, a plant-derived sweetener with zero calories, is one of the healthier sugar substitute options available today.

While added sugar has negative health consequences, artificial sweeteners are no better. In a world where we are all striving to be healthier, it's amazing that we are willing to continue to eat food with laboratory prepared, modified chemicals that cause chronic inflammation and disease.

COMMON SUGARS

- anhydrous dextrose
- brown sugar
- cane crystals
- cane sugar
- corn sweetener
- corn syrup solids
- corn syrup
- crystal dextrose
- evaporated cane juice
- fructose sweetener
- fruit juice concentrates
- high-fructose corn syrup
- honey
- liquid fructose
- malt syrup
- maple syrup
- molasses
- pancake syrup
- raw sugar
- stevia
- sugar syrup
- white sugar

LESS COMMON SUGARS

- carbitol
- concentrated fruit juice
- corn sweetener
- diglycerides
- disaccharides
- erythritol
- evaporated cane juice
- fructooligosaccharides (FOS)
- galactose
- glucitol
- glucoamine
- hexitol
- inversol
- isomalt
- malted barley
- maltodextrin
- malts
- mannitol
- nectars
- pentose
- raisin syrup
- ribose rice syrup
- rice malt
- rice syrup solids
- sorbitol
- sorghum
- sucanat
- sucanet
- xylitol
- zylose

Aspartame, sucralose, saccharin, and other "fake" sugars are all concocted in a laboratory and are not ingredients that your body is supposed to be ingesting. These artificial ingredients can cause underlying inflammation in the body that can worsen human illness, including cancer and auto-immune disease. Unfortunately, more than 6,000 grocery items, including diet drinks, yogurts, gum, and sugar free items currently contain artificial sweeteners. The list below includes some of the most common artificial sweeteners found in the foods we eat.

ARTIFICIAL SWEETENERS

- acesulfame potassium
- advantame
- alitame
- aspartame
- aspartame-acesulfame salt
- cyclamate

- glycyrrhizin
- hydrogenated starch hydrolysate (HSH)
- isomalt
- lactitol
- maltitol
- mannitol

- neohesperidin dc
- neotame
- polydextrose
- saccharin
- sorbitol
- sucralose
- tagatose

Although marketed as not contributing to weight gain and blood sugar elevations—though the jury is still out—artificial sweeteners do contribute to human disease in other ways. Do you know what *does* feed on the artificial sweeteners we consume? The bad guys in your gut microbiome! Feeding the bad guys on a regular basis increases the number of foreign bacteria, contributing to chronic inflammation and immune activation. In fact, there is some evidence that eliminating aspartame can dramatically reduce Hashimoto's antibodies in some people, though further studies need to be done. Elimination of these artificial sweeteners likely helps to decrease gut inflammation, quiets the immune response, and reduces *fighting gut*.

OUR ADVICE: The best thing to do is to eliminate added sugar and artificial sweeteners completely. If you have a craving for something sweet, go for fruit. Fresh fruit is better than fruit juice, which is higher in sugar and lower in fiber. If you do have small amounts of fruit juice, be aware that fresh squeezed fruit juice has more fiber than packaged juice. Also, fresh fruit is preferable to dried fruit, which has higher levels of sugar and calories.

■ Foe #3: Halogenated Thyroid Disrupters

Non-metallic elements, called halogens (including bromine, fluorine, and chlorine) are some of the most common thyroid disruptors—and unfortunately, are often found in our food. If you pull up a copy of the Periodic Table of Elements on the Internet, you will see that all of the halogens are stacked up on each other because they are similar in action and structure. You may notice that there is a fourth halogen in the table—iodine!

Bromides

Bromide is a halogen similar to iodide. Because the two elements are related, heavily brominated foods can compete with iodide uptake in the thyroid gland, contributing to hypothyroidism, thyroid nodules, and, likely, the development of thyroid cancer. Although many bromides are now banned, they are still present in some of our food and drinks.

In the United States, bromides were commonly found in a pesticide called methyl bromide mainly used on strawberries grown in California. Thankfully, the use of methyl bromide on American grown strawberries was banned in 2016. Still, traces of this compound may be found in foods, including grapes imported from Chile, and in certain rice, pet foods, walnuts, plums, figs, raisin, dates, and dried pork products. Instead of methyl bromide, many farmers now use chloropicrin, another toxic chemical that may also affect thyroid function.

OUR ADVICE: Buy organic strawberries and produce, particularly those fruits and vegetables that are associated with the highest pesticide residue. You may have heard of a list called the "Dirty Dozen," which includes fruits and vegetables widely believed to have the highest chemical residue. Whenever possible, buy the organic versions of these fruits and vegetables.

The Dirty Dozen

The "Environmental Working Group" found the following fruits and vegetables to have the highest levels of pesticides, based on more than 38,000 samples. They appear in descending order of pesticide contamination.

1. Strawberries	5. Grapes	9. Tomatoes
2. Spinach	6. Peaches	10. Celery
3. Nectarines	7. Cherries	11. Potatoes
4. Apples	8. Pears	12. Sweet Bell Peppers

Although we have started to crack down on methyl bromide, brominated vegetable oil (BVO) is still abundant in in citrus drinks and soft drinks, including Mountain Dew, Sun Drop, AMP Energy Drinks, and others. BVO is a flame retardant used in *rocket fuel* that just so happens to also make a handy beverage emulsifier—that is, both a preservative and food stabilizer—so, when added to drinks, it prevents flavoring from separating from the other ingredients. Another brominated compound, potassium bromate, can be found as a dough conditioner in certain commercial bakery products, wraps, rolls, breadcrumbs, bagel chips, and flour. Unfortunately, there are also numerous thyroid disruptors in the environment, many of which we'll discuss in Chapter 11.

OUR ADVICE: Don't buy brominated products, and buy organic produce for those items listed in the Dirty Dozen. Concentrate on foods with the least amount of pesticide residue, such as avocados, sweet corn, pineapples, onion, asparagus, and papayas.

Fluorides

Like bromide, fluoride can also compete with iodide uptake into the thyroid gland. Fluoride derived pesticides can be found in grape products, dried fruit, dried beans, cocoa powder, and walnuts. Tea plants can also absorb fluoride from the soil and are most highly concentrated in older tea leaves. Interestingly, green tea, which is recognized for its antioxidant properties, tends to have high amounts of fluoride. The exception is ceremonial grade matcha tea, which is grown using traditional Japanese methods and utilizes younger leaves. White tea also has lower amounts of fluoride.

Fluoride is also found in 95 percent of our toothpastes. In the 1950s, fluoride was added to public drinking water in the United States as a public health measure to protect against tooth decay. Since that time, there have been a few studies that have linked fluorinated drinking water to the development of hypothyroidism, though further research is needed.

OUR ADVICE: While you're probably okay brushing your teeth with a small amount of fluoride toothpaste, if you're concerned, there are fluoride free toothpastes available. And if you don't want to ingest fluoride in drinking water, you can avoid it by using certain water filters, or by drinking spring or distilled water.

Chlorides

Chloride, another halogen that competes with iodide, is most commonly found in table salt as sodium chloride. Research with animals shows some

How to Read a Nutrition Label

Reading nutrition labels is imperative in determining whether the products you buy are nutrient-packed or simply full of artificial ingredients and other unhealthy substances. The steps below will teach you what to look for when reading the labels and deciding which foods you should or shouldn't be eating.

Nutrition Facts	
Serving Size 24g	
Servings per Container 12	
Amount Per Serving	
Calories 140	Calories from Fat 40
	% Daily Value
Total Fat 4.5g	**7%**
Saturated Fat 0.5g	**3%**
Trans Fat 0g	
Polyunsaturated Fat 1g	
Monounsaturated Fat 2g	
Cholesterol 0g	**0%**
Sodium 0g	**0%**
Total Carbohydrate 27g	**9%**
Dietary Fiber 5g	**19%**
Sugars 0g	
Protein 5g	**0%**
Vitamin A 0% • Vitamin C 0%	
Calcium 2% • Iron 6%	

*Percent Daily Values are based on a 2,000 calorie diet. Your daily values may be higher or lower depending on your calorie needs:

	Calories:	2,000	2,500
Total Fat	Less than	65g	80g
Saturated Fat	Less than	20g	25g
Cholesterol	Less than	300mg	300mg
Sodium	Less than	2,400mg	2,400mg
Total Carbohydrate		300g	375g
Dietary Fiber		25g	30g

Calories per gram:
Fat 9 • Carbohydrate 4 • Protein 4

1. Start with the serving size, at the top of the label. Compare the amount you eat with a standard serving size, which the daily recommended allowance (RDA) is based on.

2. Be aware of the amount of sugars, saturated fats, carbohydrates, and sodium. You want to limit these. They are found in higher amounts in processed foods.

3. Look for beneficial nutrients, such as vitamins C and A, iron, fiber, potassium, iron, and calcium.

4. Use the 5 to 20 rule as a quick reference. This informal rule can serve as a guideline, with the idea being that 5 percent of the RDA for any nutrient is considered low, and 20 percent is considered high. So for the good nutrients, you want a higher percentage, and conversely, for the unhealthy ones (like saturated fats, artificial ingredients, sugars, and salt), look for a low percentage.

evidence that high salt intake can decrease thyroid hormone production in hyperthyroidism. Additional evidence points to sodium chloride reducing the strength of certain T cell soldiers, contributing to autoimmunity. These effects are separate from the effect of excess iodide in iodinated salt, something we will discuss later in Chapter 10.

OUR ADVICE: Limit salt, and if your doctor recommends iodine, get it from a multivitamin. We will discuss the iodine controversy, as well as supplements, in Chapter 10.

TABLE 9.2. TOP ANTIOXIDANT AND ANTI-INFLAMMATORY FOODS

FOOD GROUP	EXAMPLES
Beverages	Black tea, coffee, cocoa, green tea, lemon juice, organic fruit juices with no added sugar (apple, orange, and pomegranate), red tea, red wine, rosé wine.
Desserts/Fruits	Fruit, or an occasional small piece of dark chocolate (about one ounce). Acai, apple, bananas, blackberry, black chokeberry, black currant, black elderberry, black grape, grapefruit, green grape, lemon, lime, lowbush blueberry, highbush blueberry, nectarine, orange, plum, peach, prune, red currant, red raspberry, strawberry, and sweet cherry.
Herbs and Spices	Basil, capers, celery seed, ceylon cinnamon, Chinese cinnamon, cloves, curry powder, dill, dried marjoram, dried rosemary, dried sage, dried spearmint, dried thyme, dried peppermint, ginger, lemon verbena, Mexican oregano, parsley, star anise, and turmeric.
Nuts, Seeds, and Legumes	Almonds, black beans, Brazil nuts, cashews, chia seeds, chestnuts, fava beans, flaxseed, kidney beans, hazelnuts, pecan, pinto snap beans, pistachios, organic soybeans, and walnuts.
Oils	Coconut oil, extra virgin olive oil, and vinegar.
Proteins, Omega-3 Rich Fish, and Shellfish	Atlantic mackerel, catfish, chicken, freshwater trout, herring, rainbow trout, oysters, salmon, and sardines.
Vegetables	Artichokes, asparagus, beets, black olives, bok choy, broccoli, carrot, celery, curly endive, eggplant, green chicory, green olives, green onion, kale, okra, peppers, potatoes, red chicory, red lettuce, red onion, romaine lettuce, shallot, spinach, tomatoes, and yellow onion.

BEST FOODS FOR HASHIMOTO'S

So, what are the best foods to eat if you have Hashimoto's thyroiditis? Any foods that decrease inflammation in the gut and provide optimal nutrients for thyroid function. An anti-inflammatory diet rich in antioxidants and omega-3 fatty acids is ideal for optimal thyroid health.

Here are some of the best foods to eat if you have Hashimoto's disease:

- *Fresh fruits and vegetables (organic, if possible).* Focus on green leafy vegetables and berries.

- *Lean protein.* Grass-fed beef, pasture-raised chicken and turkey, and low-mercury fish, such as salmon, shrimp, tilapia, and catfish, which are all lean sources of protein.

- *Olive oil.* Nuts, such as almonds and walnuts, are also good in moderation, which is about a handful a day.

- *Fermentable foods.* These foods are a great a way of introducing good bacteria into the microbiome. Think of these as the food version of a probiotic, something we will discuss in more detail in Chapter 10. Fermented foods include kefir, komboucha, sauerkraut, homemade pickles (without vinegar), miso, tempeh, natto, and kimchi.

When considering optimal foods for someone with Hashimoto's, the best foods are the ones that have the most anti-inflammatory properties and the highest concentration of antioxidants. Think of an antioxidant as a food that works to clean up all of the debris in the body after your T and B cell soldiers are done fighting. If excess debris is left in the body, it can work as a harmful oxidizing agent that contributes to AITD symptoms and makes you sick. Table 9.2 will provide you with examples of the top antioxidants that you should freely integrate into your diet. These foods have the highest concentrations of polyphenols, flavonoids, and omega-3 fatty acids.

FOOD CONTROVERSIES ASSOCIATED WITH HASHIMOTO'S

If you have ever searched on the web for "what to eat if you have thyroid disease," you probably found an overwhelming amount of mixed information—from eliminating gluten to avoiding cruciferous vegetables to avoiding soy. It's hard to know where to start with your diet. Again, just remember, everyone is different, and there is no one-size-fits all approach. As we review the different controversies and theories related to food and Hashimoto's, be sure to work with your doctor to determine whether an elimination of any of the following foods is right for you.

■ The Gluten Controversy

For quite some time, it seems as if everybody is allergic to or intolerant to gluten. What is gluten, anyway? Gluten is the general name for the protein found in wheat products and related grains, but it can be a hidden ingredient in many other processed foods. Thankfully, the food industry has provided many gluten-free options in our grocery stores. As we discussed in Chapter 4, there is an undisputed increased risk of celiac disease in patients with Hashimoto's disease. Additionally, new studies and testing have shown that even patients who test negative for celiac disease can have gluten sensitivity, meaning that they also react poorly to gluten, but to a lesser degree. If you are gluten intolerant or have celiac disease, you should *absolutely* follow a gluten-free diet. But does *everybody* with AITD need to follow a gluten-free diet?

The evidence shows probably not. Admittedly, there have not been many good, long-term studies looking at the gluten-free diet and how it changes antibodies in Hashimoto's disease. But the evidence that does exist demonstrates that while Hashimoto's antibodies may worsen in patients that also have celiac antibodies, a gluten-free diet has no effect on Hashimoto's antibodies in patients without celiac disease or gluten sensitivity. Therefore, if you have no evidence for gluten intolerance or celiac disease, you likely do not need to follow a gluten-free diet.

Additionally, more recent studies have shown that even in patients with celiac disease, there may be no effect of a gluten-free diet in AITD disease progression. If you have questions of whether you're gluten intolerant or have celiac disease, discuss them with your doctor. If you're still not sure, it is reasonable to follow a gluten-free diet for up to four weeks and determine if your symptoms improve. It's worth noting that even in the absence of a formal celiac disease or gluten sensitivity diagnosis, some patients do notice an improvement in symptoms with gluten elimination. As we've mentioned previously, there is no one-size-fits-all approach to Hashimoto's, even when it comes to diet.

■ Dairy

Did you know that there are very few people that are actually lactose intolerant or sensitive? In reality, most people with a dairy allergy are allergic to a milk protein called casein, as opposed to whey, which is the major protein in many protein shakes and bars. Why are people allergic to casein? Because about 2,000 years ago, the normal cow milk protein, called casein A2, underwent a mutation to a new milk protein called casein A1. The result? An immune response to a foreign protein that our immune systems were not familiar with!

Casein A1 is the protein that most people with a dairy intolerance are allergic to. This explains why some people with a dairy sensitivity have no issues eating things like Italian gelato, where many of the cows are still producing the native casein A2 protein. The moral of the story? If you have a dairy intolerance, look for dairy products made from casein A2-producing cows, or avoid it altogether.

Many dietary protocols for Hashimoto's call for dairy elimination. In people who are dairy intolerant, it makes sense to eliminate dairy items that could be producing an inflammatory response in the gut. But if you have no issues with dairy, there is currently no evidence to support the idea that eliminating it will improve AITD symptoms or reduce antibodies.

■ Soy

Similar to gluten and dairy, there is a school of thought that soy may also adversely affect thyroid function. Soy is a phytoestrogen, meaning that it has estrogen-like properties in the body. Because of this, in large quantities, it can potentially alter something called thyroid binding globulin, or TBG, causing changes in thyroid hormone. Additionally, soy has been shown to influence thyroid medication absorption. Despite this, there's currently no evidence that eating soy in moderation significantly influences thyroid function. Therefore, moderate soy intake is acceptable in most AITD patients.

■ Eggs and Corn

The issue raised with eggs and corn is that some AITD patients have food intolerances to these items, causing gut inflammation and worsening autoimmunity. Now there are commercially available tests to determine food sensitivities, although testing is not perfect. If you are not allergic or sensitive to these items, they should be fine to eat with Hashimoto's. Eggs, for example, are excellent sources of iodine and other important nutrients in thyroid hormone production.

■ Lectins

Some in the health and wellness community believe that plant lectins, or proteins found in the skin and seeds of some plants, legumes, and grains, can also increase gut inflammation and autoimmunity. One common lectin that we all know? Gluten. Just like gluten sensitivity, not everyone is sensitive to lectins. One way to protect yourself if you are sensitive to lectins is to eliminate gluten, beans and legumes, and nightshade vegetables (tomatoes, zucchini, eggplant, white potatoes, peppers).

You can reduce lectin content in beans and legumes by soaking them in water. Start soaking them late in the day or early evening, changing the water a couple of times before you go to sleep. Let them soak overnight and then rinse and drain once again in the morning. Pressure cooking also helps to reduce lectins, although it is not universally effective among all lectin-rich foods (it doesn't work for gluten). Not ready to get rid of your tomatoes just yet? You can alternatively peel and de-seed your nightshade vegetables to get rid of the parts most highly concentrated with lectins.

■ Cruciferous Vegetables

Cruciferous vegetables are leafy green crops that are named for the cross-like shape of their four petals. These popular vegetables are high in vitamins, nutrients, and antioxidants. Some of the most commonly eaten cruciferous veggies include:

- arugula
- brocoli
- Brussels sprouts
- cabbage
- cauliflower
- collard greens
- horseradish
- kale
- radishes
- watercress

You can find a comprehensive list of cruciferous vegetables and more information about their health benefits online.

There is a theoretical risk that eating raw cruciferous vegetables can produce a substance called thiocyanate, which interferes with the uptake of iodide in the thyroid gland, thereby contributing to the development of goiter. The real risk? Unless you're eating ridiculously large quantities of uncooked cruciferous vegetables, there should be no real effect on your thyroid levels. Eating these items is important, as they also produce substances that inhibit the inflammatory response. Therefore, eat these raw vegetables in moderation, and as many cooked cruciferous vegetables as you like.

■ The Controversy Over Genetically Modified Organisms (GMOs)

The topic of GMOs has become a hot political debate. On one hand, GMO foods are important in feeding the world's population, but on the other hand, people continue to question the safety of GMO-related foods. A GMO is any food, beverage, or medication (insulin, for example) produced with living organisms that have been genetically modified in a laboratory. In the laboratory, foreign genes derived from bacteria, viruses, insects, animals, and even humans are inserted into the organism to make them resistant to chemicals, maintain a longer shelf life, or look more appetizing to the consumer.

GMOs are controversial, with many science and health experts of the belief that they are safe for human consumption. This includes the prestigious Academies of Science. Still, a recent study published in *Nature* demonstrated significant changes in over 150 proteins between GMO and non-GMO corn, new genetically modified molecules that may look foreign to your good bacteria and promote fighting gut. Just think about what your gut microbiome could be potentially signaling to your immune cells when they encounter these genetically altered proteins and organisms!

The most commonly genetically modified foods include corn, soy beans, tomatoes, zucchini, rapeseed, potatoes, rice, sugar beets, papayas, yellow summer squash, apples, canola oil, and dairy from cows injected with a certain type of growth hormone called r-BGH. Most packaged foods contain ingredients derived from corn, soy, canola, and sugar beet—and the vast majority of these crops grown in North America are genetically modified. Even animals that are fed soy and corn, including vegetarian-fed chicken and beef may have exposure to GMOs.

OUR ADVICE: There are a number of steps you can take to reduce your intake of GMOs. Raising your awareness level and putting some effort into what you consume will make a big difference in reducing potentially harmful GMOs:

- Look for "GMO-free" or "non-GMO" on food labels.

- Limit or eliminate foods that are classically GMO-altered. These include alfalfa, canola, corn, soy, sugar, sugar beet, yellow summer squash, and zucchini.

- Grow produce in your own garden with non-GMO seeds.

How to Read Your Produce

Do you know those little stickers on your fruits and vegetables? They are not only there to help the cashier check you out, but serve as a numbering system to determine if your food is organic, nonorganic, or GMO-modified. According to the International Federation for Produce Standards (IFPS), companies can voluntarily elect to place a price look-up code (PLU) on the food or vegetable to declare whether it is organic, not organic, or GMO-modified. The bad news? This is an entirely elective process, and GMO food companies do not need to declare their food as GMO-modified (in many European countries they do).

Here is how to interpret those little stickers.

- A **four-digit code** is standard and could mean any of the following.

- A **five-digit code** starting with the number 9 should mean organic, although you should look for that USDA-certified organic sticker to be sure.

- A **five-digit code** starting with the number 8 is used to mean GMO-modified, although GMO-modified produce can also "hide" under the four-digit codes. Now, the IFPS is using 5-digit codes starting with 83000 to signify standard produce and 84000 to signify organic produce, while entirely eliminating the code for GMO modification. If a food is organic and USDA certified, it should be non-GMO, according to USDA National Organic Standards.

ELIMINATION DIETS

Because there is no one-size-fits-all approach to diet, it is sometimes recommended that patients follow a multi-step elimination regimen. If you eliminate all of the above foods we've discussed at the same time, you won't know which one is the most important in reducing your autoimmune disease. Therefore, an elimination diet with one to two items removed at a time is sometimes recommended to follow in four to eight week intervals. If AITD antibodies improve and symptoms resolve, then you may have uncovered the diet you need to follow to optimize your own individual thyroid health and immunity. If nothing changes, feel free to reintroduce the foods you eliminated. (See inset on page 129 for instructions on how to follow a Hashimoto's elimination diet.)

Technology is actively working on how to better identify which foods you may have an intolerance to, which is different from an allergy, and which foods can activate your individual immune response. There are IgE and IgG food testing studies available, but they are not perfect and can lead to false results. The best thing to do is to follow a stepwise elimination diet to determine your individual response.

Hashimoto's Elimination Diet Protocol

Below is a stepwise elimination diet protocol to determine the effects of certain foods on Hashimoto's symptoms and antibody levels. The elimination protocol is listed in order of importance, based on population data and the overall frequency of food intolerances, but remember—everybody is different! Eliminate one food category at a time.

If eliminating a certain food improves symptoms but doesn't completely resolve them, stay off that food and eliminate the next food on the list. If there is no effect on symptoms, add that food back and eliminate the food type in the subsequent category. Keep in mind that some people are sensitive to multiple food categories.

1. Start by eliminating all the foods to avoid (see page 114) and try to stay off them for four to eight weeks, if not indefinitely. Recheck thyroid levels and antibodies after abstaining from foods on the list for at least four weeks.

2. If there is no effect, consider a trial of gluten elimination. Recheck thyroid levels and antibodies every four to eight weeks.

3. If eliminating gluten from your diet still has no impact, reintroduce gluten and eliminate dairy. Recheck thyroid levels and antibodies in four to eight weeks.

4. If you are still experiencing adverse effects of Hashimoto's, reintroduce dairy and eliminate nuts, eggs, corn, lectin, and soy, in that order. When eliminating corn, lectin, and soy, remember to buy pasture raised, grass fed, and grass finished meat, as many animals are fed corn and soybeans. Many times, animals fed corn and soybeans are still marketed as vegetarian-fed.

CONCLUSION

Finding the ideal Hashimoto's diet for you may not be an easy or quick process, but there are some immediate changes you can make to your diet to reduce or eliminate inflammation. Quieting the immune response in your gut is important in reducing the systemic autoimmune response that is driving your thyroid disease.

Processed foods are everywhere and hard to avoid. It takes mindfulness and dedication. If you're used to eating a lot of processed foods, it will probably be a challenge to make better choices. It's work, but it's also worth it. By being aware of what you consume (and avoid), you put yourself in the driver's seat of your health care. While there are certain aspects of Hashimoto's that you have no control over, food is one area where you can take command. By developing healthier eating habits, you are contributing to the betterment of your health. This is one area where *you* have the power to make a difference.

Remember, dietary changes in AITD will not result in an immediate fix. It will take time for your fighting gut to stop its attack strategy and reinstate a peaceful, non-inflammatory environment. Be persistent in your lifestyle modifications and don't give up! In addition to dietary changes, there are other vitamins and supplements that can work in a similar fashion to quiet the immune response. We will discuss all of these, in addition to optimizing your gut microbiome, in Chapter 10.

10.

Hashimoto's and Nutritional Supplements

Finding the right supplements for treating Hashimoto's can quickly become overwhelming. Because there are only a few good research trials, the vitamin, mineral, or compound recommended for you may vary considerably from practitioner to practitioner. Many of these nutrients act in similar ways, whereas others are synergistic, meaning that when they are combined, they can create an intensified effect. Being selective in the vitamins you use is of utmost importance in maintaining optimal thyroid health. Too little supplementation and your immune issues may persist; too much supplementation and you can make yourself sick in other ways.

The fact is, as consumers, we are all constantly bombarded by ads that try to sell us things by appealing to our needs—on the television, on the Internet, and on the radio. When ads are aimed at people suffering from a specific health issue, it often catches their attention. Unfortunately, at times, these products come with unfounded promises. Patients with thyroid issues, like anyone suffering with health problems, are not immune from these promotions. To ensure that you can make informed decisions about what to take and what to avoid, it's important to have as many facts as possible. In this chapter, we will discuss AITD-specific vitamins and other supplements that are important for optimization of thyroid health—as well as those to stay away from.

IMPROVING HASHIMOTO'S WITH NUTRITIONAL SUPPLEMENTS

Because the topic of nutritional supplements is one that can (and does) take up entire books, we are limiting it to the three main categories that affect Hashimoto's disease: thyroid-specific nutrients, anti-inflammatory nutrients, and antioxidant supplements. Many of the vitamins found within the same category work in similar ways. Therefore, you might not need to take everything mentioned here. Everyone reacts differently to what they put in their bodies, which is why it might take some time to figure out what's best for you.

- **Thyroid-specific nutrients.** These are nutrients that your thyroid gland needs to make and properly metabolize thyroid hormone.

- **Anti-inflammatory nutrients.** These are the nutrients important in quieting any inflammatory response in the body, allowing the immune system to "reboot" and re-learn the proper training manual.

- **Antioxidant supplements.** These are the nutrients needed to reverse the toxic effects that can appear as the result of longstanding inflammation and autoimmunity.

THYROID-SPECIFIC NUTRIENTS

Not only does the thyroid gland need iodide to function properly, it also needs additional essential vitamins, including zinc, selenium, magnesium, and iron. In the following section, we will discuss thyroid-essential vitamins in detail. Always remember to discuss your vitamins with your doctor and try to stay within the recommended daily allowance (RDA), or the optimal daily dose recommended by the Food and Nutrition Board, as taking too much of certain vitamins can make you sick.

Iodine

As previously discussed, we know that iodine is necessary for thyroid health. But too much iodine can actually be harmful. For most Hashimoto's patients, daily iodine intake within the RDA is fine. You are unlikely to ingest too much iodine within food, unless you eat large amounts of seafood, seaweed, or sushi regularly. Many commonly sold iodine supplements, however, include iodine at much higher concentrations than the RDA, which is set at 150 mcg daily for adults and 220 mcg daily for pregnant women. These high-dose iodine supplements can be toxic to the thyroid and actually worsen hypothyroidism. Therefore, when it comes to iodine, make sure you are following the recommended dosing guidelines.

The Iodine Controversy

Although we know that iodine is important for thyroid function, there is controversy on whether Americans even need to add it as a supplement because it is now so prevalent in our diet. We know that in the 1900s, iodine was added to our salt supply as a public health measure to prevent endemic goiter. The addition of iodine effectively resolved the worldwide issue of goiter. But was the addition of iodine to table salt truly a good thing?

After the introduction of iodized salt, studies around the world showed that there was also a rise in AITD, particularly an increase in thyroglobulin antibodies (TgAb). In Chapter 9, we learned that salt is composed of a chloride halogen that may interfere with our T cells and the immune system. Thus, although the addition of iodine may have resolved endemic goiter, the increased use of salt (a halogenated compound) may have contributed to the rise in thyroid autoimmunity. In addition, there are reports that too much iodine added to salt is also toxic to the thyroid. Because of conflicting data, the American Thyroid Association has prioritized research that addresses whether iodine is helpful or harmful in patients with thyroid dysfunction.

OUR ADVICE: The best way to get iodine is through iodine-rich foods, including dairy, egg yolks, small amounts of seaweed (as a food, not a supplement), and seafood, most notably shrimp. Alternatively, you can elect to supplement with low-dose iodine in your multivitamin, within the RDA amounts. Using a small amount of iodized salt, such as $1/3$ teaspoon daily, is another option. However, if you have very high levels of AITD antibodies, particularly TgAbs, you should talk to your doctor about limiting the amount of salt and iodine in your diet, or possibly eliminating them altogether.

Iron

Did you know that iron deficiency, like iodine deficiency, can also contribute to the development of thyroid goiter? This is because the thyroid needs iron for the production of thyroid hormone, particularly for the proper function of one of the main thyroid hormone-producing machines, TPO. Iron has also been shown to improve iodide uptake from the blood and helps with T4 to T3 conversion. If you are iron deficient, you may have many of the same symptoms that you get when you're hypothyroid. These include:

- Chronic fatigue and low energy
- Exercise intolerance
- Difficulty staying warm
- Hair loss or lack of growth

OUR ADVICE: Work with your doctor to figure out if you are iron deficient. There are many available forms of iron supplementation. Be aware that frequent side effects from iron supplements include black stools and upset stomach. Because of this, work closely with your doctor to find the formulation that works best for you.

Magnesium

Magnesium can affect thyroid function in multiple ways. It's needed for the thyroid to effectively pick up iodide from the blood and make thyroid hormone. It also works to enhance DIO in the conversion of T4 to T3. The thyroid gland not only needs magnesium to produce adequate thyroid hormone, but magnesium sulfate also contributes to anti-inflammatory processes important in quieting the immune response. Magnesium comes in many different forms, but magnesium citrate, magnesium glycinate, and magnesium malate generally have the best absorption.

OUR ADVICE: Take a magnesium supplement, if needed, in recommended amounts. (See Table 10.1 on page 142.) Magnesium is also found in green leafy vegetables, such as spinach, and in legumes, nuts, seeds, and whole grains.

■ Selenium

Selenium is one of the most important minerals in autoimmune thyroid disease. In fact, the thyroid is the organ with the highest concentration of selenium in the body. Selenium works in multiple ways to optimize your thyroid function and calm your immune response.

Specifically, it works by:

- Decreasing inflammation
- Improving DIO function and optimizing the conversion of T4 to T3 (DIO needs selenium to function properly)
- Promoting peaceful T cells, thereby decreasing autoimmunity

- Reducing both TPO and TG antibodies with time

- Supporting antioxidant enzymes that protect the worker bee thyroid cells from harm

What a great mineral! There are multiple research studies that support the use of selenium in AITD. In fact, most studies demonstrate about a 40 percent reduction in AITD antibodies after three to four months of being on the vitamin. The jury is still out on what this means for AITD symptoms and thyroid function, but it's reasonable to think that decreasing the immune response against the thyroid most likely also decreases thyroid gland destruction. Interestingly, selenium has also been shown to significantly improve Graves' eye disease in hyperthyroid patients by reducing Graves' antibodies and the immune response.

OUR ADVICE: Selenium can usually be found in your multivitamin at concentrations of 50 micrograms to 100 micrograms daily, although we recommend that AITD patients go higher. (See Table 10.1 on page 142.)

A word of caution: Do not take over 400 micrograms of selenium daily, because in large amounts selenium can be toxic. Another way to get selenium is through Brazil nuts, though the selenium concentration in the nut depends on the soil concentration in which it was grown. Check labels or ask the manufacturer how much selenium is in a serving of their Brazil nuts. Other food sources of selenium include oysters, tuna, whole-wheat bread, sunflower seeds, mushrooms, and rye.

Zinc and Copper

We have grouped zinc and copper together because they work in a seesaw relationship. If you have too much zinc in the body, you can deplete your copper stores, and vice versa. Both elements, but particularly zinc, are important in maintaining proper thyroid function. Because both minerals are vital thyroid-specific nutrients, it is important that they are balanced. Like selenium, zinc works in multiple ways to enhance thyroid metabolism:

- It helps with T4 to T3 conversion and maintaining healthy T3 levels

- It improves memory loss and brain fog

- It maintains normal resting metabolic rate (or weight)
- It prevents excess hair loss in hypothyroidism
- It promotes healthy signaling from the pituitary gland to the thyroid

Zinc supplementation is important in hypothyroidism, but can actually worsen hyperthyroidism.

OUR ADVICE: Many multivitamins have both minerals included for proper balance. Since you should not take more than 30 mg of zinc, you might need to cut a larger dose in half or take it every other day. While oysters contain more zinc than any other food, it can also be found in red meat, poultry, beans, nuts, crab, lobster, whole grains, and dairy products.

In addition, some thyroid-specific supplement concentrations in a multivitamin may not meet the recommended daily allowance or RDA. Certain supplements, including iron, aren't always included in multivitamins. In this case, simply add that supplement as a separate pill. Make sure that the total supplement dosage does not exceed the recommended total RDA. Some patients take these thyroid-specific vitamins separately. Remember, too much of a good thing can make you sick, so stick to the RDA.

ANTI-INFLAMMATORY NUTRIENTS

The second major group of nutrients needed in AITD work primarily on the immune system. In previous chapters, we have learned that the T and B cell soldiers are working overtime with autoimmune diseases. Their continued work in AITD is driven by continued inflammatory signals that get them to stand up and fight. Therefore, one other way that we can impact the immune response in Hashimoto's thyroiditis is by decreasing inflammation. Luckily, there are anti-inflammatory vitamins available that have this effect.

Vitamin A

Vitamin A works primarily on the immune system to regulate T and B cells and reduce the inflammatory response. Low vitamin A levels contribute to fighting gut and the breakdown of the stonewall. In addition to its anti-inflammatory properties, studies have suggested that vitamin A is important in optimizing T4 to T3 conversion and lowering the TSH level. In addition, vitamin A may be important in quieting the B cell snipers that produce Hashimoto's antibodies.

OUR ADVICE: Vitamin A supplementation is important in thyroid hormone regulation and modulation of the immune/inflammatory response. Vitamin A supplementation is typically found in its inactive form, retinol or beta-carotene, and is converted in the body to all-trans-retinoic acid (ATRA), the active form.

Too much vitamin A can also contribute to a high blood calcium level and cause illness. To prevent this, the FDA is requiring all future vitamin A supplements to be listed in retinol activity equivalents (RAE) units for ease of dosing, though many vitamin companies still list the dose in International Units (IU). Alternatively, vitamin A can be found in liver, fish oil, dairy, carrots, broccoli, cantaloupe, and squash. (See Table 10.1 on page 142.)

Vitamin D

Vitamin D is one of the most important vitamins in AITD. You may be thinking, "But I thought vitamin D was used for bone health. What does it have to do with my thyroid?" The answer is *everything*. Vitamin D works not only to help re-train your T and B cell soldiers, but it also helps to quiet the body's prolonged inflammatory response. Because it proverbially kills two birds with one stone, Vitamin D is essential in AITD. In addition, lower vitamin D levels are associated with more severe AITD. The reverse is also true, in that increasing vitamin D has been shown to decrease TPO antibodies and quiet the autoimmune response.

Vitamin D supplementation comes in two major forms: cholecalciferol (D$_3$) and ergocalciferol (D$_2$). Once vitamin D is processed in your liver and kidneys, it's converted into calcitriol, its active form. Calcitriol regulates the immune cells and decreases inflammatory signaling. In addition to vitamin supplements, you can get vitamin D through sun exposure or through vitamin D-rich foods like salmon, tuna, mackerel, and fish liver oil.

OUR ADVICE: The Institute of Medicine (IOM) has recommended an upper limit of 4,000 IUs of vitamin D$_3$ daily for adults. It's important to get vitamin D levels up into the mid normal range. For dosage recommendations, see Table 10.1 on page 142. Be aware, however, that individuals who have high blood calcium (known as hypercalcemia), which is related to several conditions, including sarcoidosis, tuberculosis, and certain cancers, should not take supplemental vitamin D.

Natural Oils

Certain compounds found in natural oils have established anti-inflammatory effects and can be useful in patients with AITD. Listed below are two of the most commonly cited in autoimmune thyroid disease: black cumin oil and fish oil.

Black Cumin Oil

Black cumin, or black seed oil, is derived from a flowering plant native to eastern Asia called *Nigella sativa*. Its major active ingredient, thymoquinone (TQ), has been shown to regulate the immune system and decrease inflammation. There's also evidence that black cumin powder of 2 grams/day can decrease TPO antibodies by 50 percent and improve free T3 levels in patients with Hashimoto's thyroiditis. Studies also demonstrated the benefit of black cumin oil for other autoimmune diseases, including vitiligo, a skin disorder, as well as in rheumatoid arthritis for joint pain.

OUR ADVICE: Consider using black cumin oil in a salad dressing, or using black cumin powder as a seasoning or in a smoothie. There are also pill forms available.

Fish/Krill Oil (EPA/DHA)

Eicosapentaenoic acid (EPA) and docosahexaenoic acid (DHA) are omega-3 fatty acids found in oily fish and fish oil supplements. They have multiple anti-inflammatory properties in the body that work to quiet the immune response. The utility of fish oil is well documented in autoimmune diseases like rheumatoid arthritis, lupus, and Crohn's disease. Another source of EPA and DHA, which has been steadily gaining in popularity, is krill oil. Krill are tiny crustaceans that are found in cold Antarctic waters. Krill has higher bioavailability because the omegas are delivered in phospholipid form, while the omegas in fish oil are in triglyceride form. Phospholipids are part of cells that are more easily recognized by the body than triglycerides. Krill also contains an antioxidant called astaxanthin.

Unfortunately, there have been very few studies looking at the effect of EPA/DHA on AITD, although several have reported lower Hashimoto's antibodies in pregnant women consuming a diet rich in omega-3 fatty acids. Dietary sources of omega-3 fatty acids include oily fish, chia seeds, flaxseed, hemp, and walnuts.

OUR ADVICE: Eat low-mercury, high-omega-3 oily fish, such as sardines, herring, anchovies, and mackerel; and omega-3-rich seeds and nuts; or supplement with 2 to 4 g of highly concentrated quality fish oil daily.

And remember, chronic inflammation can worsen Hashimoto's disease. The supplements we have discussed above should help to decrease inflammation, which reduces attacks on the immune system. When the immune system isn't triggered, Hashimoto's symptoms won't flare up as much.

ANTIOXIDANT SUPPLEMENTS

The third and final class of nutrients in AITD includes the antioxidants. What exactly are antioxidants, anyway, and how are they different from anti-inflammatory nutrients? Antioxidants are substances that prevent oxidation in the body. Oxidation is a damaging process caused by molecules called *free radicals*. Think of free radicals as the debris found in the body during and after the T and B cell soldiers go to war. All of this debris can accumulate in the body, contributing to fatigue and illness.

There is some overlap between anti-inflammatory and antioxidant nutrients. For example, selenium and vitamin A are not only good thyroid-specific and anti-inflammatory vitamins, but are also excellent antioxidants. However there are specific antioxidant nutrients that are *experts* at cleaning up the debris. In long-standing Hashimoto's, antioxidant nutrients are important in optimizing energy levels and decreasing autoimmunity.

Glutathione

Glutathione is a major intracellular antioxidant that works to decrease inflammation markers and reduce oxidative stress. In AITD, glutathione is needed to protect the thyroid cells from damage and oxidative stress. Unlike the above antioxidants, glutathione is not primarily found in food, but instead is made by the body. Selenium is also very important for proper glutathione peroxidase function. It's difficult to supplement glutathione, because even high dose supplemental glutathione is broken down into amino acids in the gut before being absorbed. However, research seems to indicate that supplementation with glutathione for six months can help to significantly increase body stores, so it may be worth the effort.

OUR ADVICE: Since you don't get glutathione in the diet, consider supplementing, since it is one of the most important antioxidants needed for thyroid function. Liposomal glutathione supplements are thought to be better absorbed by the body with usual dosing of one capsule twice daily. For specifics on dosing, refer to Table 10.1 on page 142. If you take glutathione, make sure to also take zinc, as long-term glutathione supplementation can reduce your zinc levels.

N-acetylcysteine (NAC)

N-acetylcysteine, or NAC, helps to boost glutathione. Like glutathione, it works to protect your thyroid worker bees from oxidative stress and damage. Unfortunately, it has common side effects of nausea, vomiting, diarrhea, and constipation, so be aware of the amount you consume at one time. Still, it can work synergistically with glutathione in preventing thyroid cell destruction.

OUR ADVICE: It is reasonable to consider adding NAC to glutathione to optimize thyroid protection against oxidative stress. If you do elect to add NAC, it is best to break it up into several doses, to make it more tolerable. For dosage amounts, refer to Table 10.1 on page 142.

Vitamin B_1

Vitamin B_1, also known as thiamine, has many important properties, including antioxidant effects. In severe illness, thiamine deficiency has been linked to increased oxidative stress and inflammation in the body. In Hashimoto's thyroiditis, it has been suggested that high-dose thiamine of 600 mg per day improves fatigue in AITD. This is likely due by its ability to reduce oxidative stress and to clean up the debris left by the fighting T and B cells. Thiamine levels may be especially low in people who regularly drink alcohol or are on the diuretic drug Lasix.

OUR ADVICE: Consider adding B_1 to your vitamin regimen. Because it's water soluble, it's hard to take too much. The extra will just come out in your urine. Therefore, it is reasonable to try a higher dosage of thiamine of 100 to 600 mg per day, for several months, in order to replete body stores and then reduce to the RDA. Food sources of thiamine include whole grains, meat, and fish, though heating food decreases its thiamine content.

Vitamin C

Vitamin C, also known as ascorbic acid, isn't just for helping when you have a cold. It's a robust antioxidant that can decrease oxidative stress—a cell-damaging condition that is the result of too many free radicals. Oxidative stress is linked with disease in Hashimoto's patients. Studies have shown that vitamin C stabilizes T cell soldiers to prevent a continued autoimmune attack. Additional studies have revealed that vitamin C lessens oxidative stress after radioactive iodine therapy in patients with thyroid cancer (discussed in Chapter 13).

OUR ADVICE: Consider adding vitamin C in the form of a daily multivitamin. Good food sources include citrus fruit, tomato, potato, red and green peppers, kiwi, broccoli, strawberries, Brussels sprouts, and cantaloupe. Consult Table 10.1 on page 142 for recommended dosages.

Vitamin E

Vitamin E, also known as alpha-tocopherol, is an excellent antioxidant. In addition to decreasing oxidative stress and calming the T cell soldier response, vitamin E has also been shown to decrease oxidative stress in the brains of people with hypothyroidism; protect the worker bee thyroid follicular cells from death; and protect the heart, muscle, and bone from long-standing oxidative stress in hyperthyroidism.

Antioxidant nutrients are among the most important vitamins in quieting the autoimmune response in AITD. Because they work to "clean up the debris" from the ongoing immune war, they can also significantly improve energy levels and well-being.

OUR ADVICE: Consider adding vitamin E into your multivitamin or vitamin regimen. Vitamin E can have some toxic effects if you take too much. Nuts, seeds, and leafy greens are the best food sources of vitamin E. Refer to Table 10.1 on page 142 for recommended dosages.

HASHIMOTO'S SUPPLEMENTS AND DOSAGES

Now that we have reviewed the most important supplements in Hashimoto's disease, we will outline the recommended dosing. Below we have listed all recommended nutrients and supplements for Hashimoto's patients in an easy-to-follow table with associated RDA dosages and safety limits. It is necessary to understand the way the amounts are referenced, because not all measurement units are the same. When you read labels, make sure that are aware of how much of an ingredient in the nutrients or supplements you take.

Here are the most common measurements terms and their abbreviations:

- IU—international units
- mcg—micrograms
- mg—milligrams
- RAE—retinol activity equivalents

TABLE 10.1. NUTRIENTS & SUPPLEMENTS FOR HASHIMOTO'S PATIENTS	
SUPPLEMENT	OUR RECOMMENDATION PER DAY
Black Cumin Oil or Powder	2 g
Copper	2 mg maximum
Fish Oil (EPA/DHA)	2 to 4 g
Glutathione	250 to 500 mg, twice a day
Iodine	150 mcg for adults and 220 mcg in pregnant females
Iron	Discuss with your doctor
Magnesium	310 to 420 mg
N-acetylcysteine (NAC)	1.2 to 2.4 g, divided into two or three daily doses for tolerability
Selenium	200 to 400 mcg
Vitamin A	700 to 900 mcg RAE or up to 5000 IU
Vitamin B1 (Thiamine)	100 to 600 mg
Vitamin C (Ascorbic Acid)	75 mg in females, 85 mg in pregnant females, 90 mg in males, and 120 mg in breast-feeding women. Maximum daily dose is 2,000 mg
Vitamin D3	1,000 to 4,000 IU
Vitamin E (alpha-tocopherol)	20 to 35 IU is recommended. Maximum daily dose is 1,000 mg or 1,500 IU
Zinc	30 mg maximum

Three Easy Steps for Adding Vitamins in Hashimoto's Disease

There are three easy steps to get the thyroid-specific vitamins you need without breaking the bank or adding another ten to fifteen pills to your regimen:

✓ **Step 1:** Add a high quality multivitamin that includes appropriate amounts of selenium, zinc, magnesium (+/– low-dose iodine, iron, copper), vitamin D_3, vitamin A, vitamin B_1, vitamin C, and vitamin E. If the multivitamin doesn't have enough of a certain substance, you may need to add additional supplements.

✓ **Step 2:** Add high quality, concentrated fish oil or black cumin oil.

✓ **Step 3:** Add liposomal glutathione or NAC.

In addition to these AITD specific vitamins, it is also important to work with your doctor to make sure that you do not have other vitamin deficiencies, such as a vitamin B_{12} deficiency that can lead to additional symptoms and worsen fatigue.

INVESTIGATIONAL SUPPLEMENTS IN HASHIMOTO'S

The jury is still out on the following vitamins, drugs, and herbal supplements for treating Hashimoto's, but we wanted to address them, as they are frequently mentioned in the thyroid community. Use caution with these particular supplements. Just because they may be promoted online, doesn't mean that they are without risk or potential problems.

Alpha-Lipoic Acid (ALA)

Alpha-Lipoic acid (ALA) is another type of omega-3 fatty acid important in decreasing inflammation. In several small studies, it has been shown to protect the thyroid from destructive effects of radiation treatment, a known contributor to hypothyroidism and thyroid cancer. In other studies, however, it contributed to hypothyroidism by preventing conversion of T4 to T3. If you decide to take this supplement, the usual dosage is 600 to 1200 mg daily. Always inform your doctor if your supplements change as changes may impact thyroid replacement dosing.

Ashwagandha Root

There are very few studies on ashwagandha root with regard to AITD, but preliminary data does suggest that it may improve serum T4 and T3. Ashwagandha root likely improves thyroid function by working as an antioxidant. While there are patients who respond well to ashwagandha, others do not find improvement and experience digestive side effects. If you decide to take this supplement, the usual dosage is 1000 to 1500 mg daily.

Curcumin (Turmeric)

Although an excellent anti-inflammatory vitamin, there is no good study that demonstrates a direct impact of curcumin on thyroid function. There is some data that curcumin may have a protective effect during radioactive iodine therapy for people with thyroid cancer. If you decide to take this supplement, you can dose it in two ways. One, as curcumin 0.5 to 7.5 grams daily divided into three to four doses. Two, as turmeric, which is a spice that contains curcumin, at 2,000 mg maximum daily in pill form or as a cooking spice measured at $1/_2$ teaspoon to $1^1/_2$ teaspoons daily.

Low-Dose Naltrexone (LDN)

Naltrexone is an opiate receptor antagonist, which means that it blocks the effects of opioids. This drug is conventionally used in high doses to counteract alcohol and opioid dependency. Conversely, low-dose naltrexone (LDN) acts as an anti-inflammatory agent and pain reliever through a non-opioid receptor on immune cells. It has been shown to be most effective in Crohn's disease, but convincing data is still lacking for AITD. Doses range from 1.5 mg to 4.5 mg daily at bedtime and typically need to be prescribed by a doctor.

Milk Thistle

Milk thistle is an herb thought to prevent glutathione depletion in patients with Hashimoto's. Unfortunately, there are some reports that silychristin, a derivative from milk thistle, actually inhibits thyroid uptake into bodily cells. If you choose to take milk thistle, the typical dose is 140 mg three times a day. Make sure you discuss this with your doctor, as it can affect thyroid medicine dosing.

Polyphenols

We mentioned polyphenols in the previous chapter on diet in Hashimoto's. Polyphenols are mainly natural antioxidants that can be found in herbal teas and berries, such as acai, black chokeberry, and black elderberry. Resveratrol is a polyphenol, for example, found in grapes, berries, and wine. Although polyphenols as a group have beneficial antioxidant properties, there is one that may not be a good fit for Hashimoto's patients—resveratrol. Resveratrol, specifically, has been shown to disrupt T4 to T3 conversion and contribute to goiter, although definitive studies still need to be performed. There are highly concentrated polyphenol powders and supplements available, though no dosing recommendation has been established. Alternatively, you can get polyphenols through berries and herbal teas in your diet as previously discussed.

Because our scientific understanding of these supplements is always changing, it is important to keep an open dialogue with your physician regarding new knowledge in how various supplements may affect thyroid function.

Thyroid Quick Tip: Taking a laundry list of vitamins isn't always beneficial to your thyroid health. Like medications, vitamins interact with each other and sometimes negatively influence thyroid hormone metabolism. Therefore, be very selective in the vitamins that you choose to take, and always bring an updated list of your vitamins and herbal supplements (including dosages) to your doctor's visit for comprehensive review.

OPTIMIZING YOUR MICROBIOME USING PROBIOTICS

In Chapter 9, we discussed how your "good guy" microbiome signals to your T and B cell soldiers to keep peace at the gut wall. We also mentioned that "bad guy" bacteria, viruses, and fungi can take over the good guy bacteria in a process called dysbiosis—meaning imbalance between the bad guy and good guy bacteria. When this occurs, T and B cell soldiers start to get signals that "all is not well" beyond the gut wall, and fighting gut develops. So what causes dysbiosis? We previously mentioned that

Allison's Experience: Dealing with Deficiencies

Long before I was diagnosed with Hashimoto's, I was dealing with certain vitamin and mineral deficiencies. For as long as I can remember, blood tests would reveal a lack of vitamin D, vitamin B_{12}, and iron. Once I had Hashimoto's, I learned that I also needed selenium.

It's been a challenge to get my levels where the need to be, and it's something that requires awareness and attention on my part—as it does for any Hashimoto's patient who needs supplementation. In my case, it wasn't always as simple as taking a pill. Trial and error has been my method, and I'm now in a place where my numbers are in the normal range.

My areas of deficiencies are common among those who suffer from hypothyroidism, whether or not they have AITD. What worked for me may not work for you, but since we probably have some shared obstacles in this area, I'll explain what has worked for me.

Getting my vitamin B_{12} up was something I just couldn't do. I took oral supplements. I tried injections administered monthly at a doctor's office, and later on, weekly shots I did myself. Neither moved my number significantly. Eventually, I found out I had a genetic mutation called MTHFR. It's believed that 30 to 50 percent of the population has the mutation. So while it's somewhat common, it's controversial and beyond the scope of this book. I mention it because the mutation made it impossible for me to absorb B_{12} except in methylated form. So I tried a methyl B_{12}, also called methylcobalamin. It worked relatively quickly and has kept my levels normal.

artificial sweeteners and processed foods contribute to this imbalance, but there are other causes as well.

Medications, such as proton pump inhibitors (PPIs), including Nexium, Protonix, and Prilosec, work to lower stomach acid and are helpful for indigestion, but allow bad guy microbes to pass through the stomach, instead of killing them with stomach acid. Additional medications, such as birth control pills, ibuprofen and other NSAIDs, hand sanitizers, and frequent antibiotic use kill good guy bacteria and allow the bad guys to take over. In addition to limiting these medications and eating fresh, vitamin-rich foods, you can also optimize your microbiome by taking supplements containing a probiotic, a prebiotic, or both.

Let's move on to vitamin D. I can feel when my levels are low. My muscle pain increases and I have less energy. Conventional vitamin D supplements are typically derived from sheep lanolin, or wool grease, but not everyone reacts well to it. It made me feel sick, so I tried vegetarian vitamin D, which is derived from lichen, a plantlike organism. It comes in liquid and gummies, and is more expensive than the lanolin form. For me, it took a while to work, but my numbers increased to the normal range after a couple of months.

Iron is another problem for me. I don't eat red meat, which, in combination with my medical issues, creates an iron deficiency. For this, I use a prescription called Integra, which is similar to a prenatal vitamin. It's not covered by insurance, because it's not FDA approved (remember our discussion in Chapter 8).

As for selenium, I didn't want to add another pill to my regimen, so I researched natural ways to obtain it. I found that Brazil nuts are rich in selenium, and I now eat two to three a day. Since there's no way to test selenium levels, I go by how I'm feeling. I know that I feel better, overall, when I'm keeping up on my selenium intake by consuming Brazil nuts. Of course, every brand of Brazil nuts is sourced from different areas and carries varying amounts of selenium. Do some research when selecting a brand that is right for you.

Because we aren't a one-size-fits-all group of thyroid patients, we need doctors who are willing to work with us to figure out what works best. For me, that is Dr. Henderson, but it's important that all of us have a strong doctor-patient relationship with someone who takes our individual needs into consideration.

Which Probiotics?

Probiotics are supplements packed full of good guy bacteria. Research is underway in determining how impactful probiotics can be in maintaining gut health and reducing autoimmunity. Thus far, researchers have concentrated on good guy bacteria belonging to the groups of *Lactobacillus* and *Bifidobacterium*, both of which have many strains. Studies have demonstrated a variety of possible benefits, including decreased systemic inflammation, reduced intestinal symptoms, lower blood sugar, and weight loss. Other research has raised the theoretical risk that certain strains of probiotics may increase AITD antibodies, because some strains appear somewhat similar to TPO and Tg, two of the major machines at the thyroid factory that the immune system attacks.

Prebiotics are indigestible fiber supplements that help probiotics to do their job. These are best introduced after taking probiotics for several months. If prebiotics are introduced too quickly when the bad guys still outnumber the good guys, the prebiotic food can paradoxically feed the bad guys, allowing them to grow instead. Therefore, use prebiotics, but only after you have introduced good guy bacteria to the gut for a period of time.

OUR ADVICE: There is not enough research yet to determine which probiotic strains are most beneficial in AITD and fighting gut. Therefore, look for a high-quality probiotic supplement with at least ten strains and a concentration of 20 billion colony-forming units (CFU) or above. This information is on the label. Make sure you refrigerate your probiotic, if indicated.

Consider checking your AITD antibodies six to eight weeks after starting a new probiotic to determine if there is any significant increase, indicating a cross-reaction. In this case, stop the probiotic and consider a supplement with different bacterial strains. The benefits of a probiotic supplement typically outweigh any theoretical increase in AITD antibodies. Alternatively, adding fermentable foods high in natural probiotics can also improve gut health and autoimmunity.

SELECTING HIGH QUALITY SUPPLEMENTS

Dietary supplements are not regulated by the FDA in the same way prescription drugs are, although the FDA does have the ability to stop companies from selling their products if found to be unsafe. This is done only *after* harm has been caused, which is why it's up to the consumer to ensure they are taking a high quality supplement. Remember that more is *not* necessarily better when it comes to supplements. Just like people respond differently to prescriptions, they also respond differently to supplements. Even though a prescription is not needed for nutritional supplements and they are overall considered safe, side effects can still occur. Always look at the labels when searching for a supplement, because a lot of pertinent information can be found there. Look for the following information:

- GMP (Good Manufacturing Practices) certified.

- Limit possible allergens, such as dairy, soy or gluten.

- Look for plant-based supplements marked "Organically Certified," meaning that they are grown in soil without synthetic fertilizers or pesticides.

- No added color, sugar, or artificial flavor.

- No fillers

- No GMOs

- No growth hormones

Higher quality brands use ingredients with greater bioavailability, meaning more of the nutrient gets absorbed by your body. They also do research on their products, which can usually be found on the company website. And while an expensive price tag doesn't always equate with a better product, higher quality ingredients are normally more expensive—typically resulting in a pricier product than a discount store brand. Still, you can buy most higher priced supplements at discounted prices if you shop around.

HASHIMOTO'S AND CAUTIONARY SUPPLEMENTS

While there are many helpful supplemental options for Hashimoto's patients, there are others that must be approached with caution. Certain nutritional supplements can actually be harmful and worsen your condition. There are people admitted to hospitals every day because of problems due to supplements, either because they take too much of something, mix supplements together, or take supplements that interact with their prescriptions. We will go over the most common ones that you should avoid.

Biotin

Although Hashimoto's patients do not have to refrain from using biotin, they need to be aware that it can cause false thyroid lab readings. Biotin has been known to cause falsely elevated thyroid hormone levels, which could impact thyroid care. For this reason, you should not take biotin for at least 48 hours prior to thyroid testing.

Licorice Root (*Glycyrrhiza glabra*)

Many Hashimoto's patients supplement with adrenal boosters or licorice root to address a problem called *adrenal fatigue*, which we will discuss in further detail in Chapter 12. Although some of these products are not harmful, taking high-dose licorice root can actually cause severe health issues, including increased blood pressure, muscle weakness, low potassium, and abdominal weight gain. Therefore, if you choose to take licorice root, you should do so in moderation.

Thyroid Glandulars

Many thyroid glandular products are hidden in over-the-counter thyroid boosters and thyroid support vitamins. Like prescription-gland desiccated pig thyroid (Armour, Nature-throid), these unregulated supplements contain desiccated cow thyroid gland, which is usually listed as "bovine thyroid extract." Many of these manufacturers do not regulate the amount of thyroid hormone contained in their product. Therefore, Hashimoto's patients can be unknowingly exposed to toxic amounts of thyroid medicine if they take thyroid boosters in addition to their thyroid replacement medication. Too much thyroid hormone can cause hyperthyroid symptoms and lead to heart issues and other medical conditions. This is another reason to be sure that you review all of your supplements with your doctor.

CONCLUSION

The right supplements can be a useful and effective tool in your Hashimoto's care. Be an informed and responsible consumer when you consider adding any supplements. It's important to be informed about your choices, which includes knowing who produces the supplement, what is a safe dose, and whether or not it can interfere with other medicines or lab test results. Ideally, patients should provide an updated list of their supplements, including manufacturer and dosages, at all of their doctor visits. Your pharmacist is another helpful resource when it comes to discussing supplementation.

Remember that marketing techniques can be misleading. Just because something is advertised as *healthy* or *natural* doesn't mean it is. Not all supplements enhance thyroid function, and as we've discussed, some actually negatively affect thyroid health. Always work with your doctor to determine the supplement plan that is right for you.

Although nutritional deficiencies can contribute to autoimmunity and thyroid dysfunction, there are other, more sinister environmental toxins that are harder to avoid. We will next explore how environmental exposures also contribute to autoimmunity and what you can do to avoid them.

II.

Environmental Exposures and Hashimoto's

As we now know, AITD is influenced by a variety of different factors. So far, we have discussed the impact of genetics and nutritional status on T and B cell soldier regulation. In Chapter 3, we also mentioned that Hashimoto's thyroiditis is usually triggered by some kind of precipitating event, such as infections, stress, or toxic exposures. Here, we will discuss these environmental triggers to learn what they are, and give suggestions on how to avoid them. Reducing environmental exposures in an effort to decrease inflammation and quiet the autoimmune response is another important piece of the puzzle in improving AITD.

In Hashimoto's and other types of thyroid disease, like thyroid cancer, there are three main types of environmental exposures:

- **Infections.** This includes primarily viral but also some bacterial and fungal infections.

- **Drugs.** This includes over-the-counter and prescription medicines.

- **Pollutants and allergens.** This includes exposure to airborne allergens, skin irritants, environmental toxins, and synthetic chemicals.

In this chapter, you will find some of the most common Hashimoto's triggers, with tips on how to avoid exposure and improve thyroid health.

COMMON INFECTIONS FOUND WITH HASHIMOTO'S

Viruses, bacteria, and fungi are all around us. They live in animals and insects, on our foods, and essentially on the surfaces of everything we touch. Often times, they are also transferred through the very air we breathe. There are several organisms that cause disease, called pathogens, which have been strongly associated with the onset of AITD. Once exposed, these infectious triggers can send the T and B cell soldiers into fight mode, contributing to the development of autoimmunity. All infectious triggers share common effects—they stimulate the immune system and increase inflammation. When the immune system is triggered strongly enough, AITD can occur.

Here are the most common pathogens associated with AITD, along with the most commonly used interventions to reduce your exposure.

■ Viral Infections

Human Herpesvirus-6 (HHV-6) and Epstein-Barr Virus (EBV or HHV-4) are the two most commonly cited, but not the only, viruses associated with Hashimoto's disease. Both of these viruses are members of the herpes virus family and are rampant in the U.S. population. In fact, up to 90 percent of Americans have been previously exposed to EBV, more commonly known as "mono." Both viruses are common in children and teenagers, but can also occur in adults. They are passed in human saliva and bodily fluids—which explains why EBV is known as "the kissing disease." Both diseases are characterized by extreme fatigue, fever, swollen lymph nodes, and rash. Still, many people who are exposed *never* get symptoms. Once exposed, both viruses remain latent within the body (hiding within cells of the immune system, likely in the bone marrow) for the rest of the person's life.

Both EBV and HHV-6 are strongly associated with the development of AITD and other diseases. There are many additional viruses that can also trigger the development of AITD. For a full list, see page 36 in Chapter 3. In addition, even if you already have had a viral exposure as a likely trigger for your AITD, exposure to yet another viral infection can worsen your thyroid disease. Unfortunately, once exposed, there is no good way to treat or remove the viral particles hiding in your body.

If you are lucky and have been not been exposed to these viruses, there are some steps you can take to prevent future exposure or re-infection.

- Make sure you wash your hands often with soap and water, particularly if you are exposed to someone who is sick. Sometimes soap doesn't kill viral particles that are on your hands. In this case, hand sanitizer may work better. Use hand sanitizer only when absolutely necessary, as frequent use can reduce the good guys in your microbiome.

- Do not share utensils or drinks with someone who is sick. Additionally, many viral infections can be active without obvious symptoms. Therefore, it is best to always use your own eating and drinking utensils.

- Make sure that you aren't kissing or intimate with someone who is actively infected.

- Limit exposure to friends or family members who are coughing, sneezing, or blowing their nose. Regularly sanitize doorknobs and toys.

With regard to viral treatment, there are no good prescription antiviral medications with action against EBV or HHV-6, although studies are ongoing. Because of the prevalence of these viruses, there are ongoing efforts to establish a vaccine.

Herbal Remedies

In the world of complementary medicine, there are several herbal remedies that have been used to assist the immune system in fighting off these latent (hidden) viral infections. While these herbs have sometimes been recommended as treatment, there still needs to be more scientific data to support their use. The most commonly used herbal remedies include:

- Astragalus membranaceus (Chinese herb)
- Berberine
- Echinacea
- Olive leaf extract
- Passionflower
- Saururus chinensis (Chinese herb)
- Thymoquinone
- Turmeric

If you've already had exposure to EBV, HHV-6, or other common viral infections, there are some things that you can do to prevent reactivation of the virus. We will discuss this in further detail in the next chapter when we talk about reducing Hashimoto's flares.

■ *H. pylori*

Another common infectious trigger associated with development of AITD is a bacteria called *H. pylori* (short for *Helicobacter pylori*). More than 50 percent of the world's population has *H. pylori* bacteria residing within their stomach cavities. Despite this, over 85 percent of people infected have no symptoms. The other 15 percent typically experience stomach pain and bleeding ulcers.

It still remains unclear how *H. pylori* infects people, but it is thought that infection is passed through saliva and contaminated food or water. Research shows that people infected with *H. pylori* are twice as likely to have AITD as people without *H. pylori*. Some studies suggest that *H. pylori* infection increases the risk for Graves' disease, but not for Hashimoto's. Nevertheless, there are some steps you can take to reduce exposure and treat an underlying infection.

- Avoid water that is not purified or treated.

- Don't eat undercooked meats or poorly washed produce.

- If you have a family member with an *H. pylori* infection, make sure that they have their own set of utensils, toothbrush, or cups. Alternatively, their items should be washed with soap and hot boiling water. Once they are treated for the infection, they can start using shared silverware again. Limit kissing and bodily fluid exposure with them while they are infected.

- Wash your hands after bathroom use and before eating your food. Make sure that your family members do the same.

- When you go out to a restaurant, make sure that you are at an establishment that requires employees to wash their hands when making and serving your food.

Because *H. pylori* infection is so common, it is easy to test for in the blood or stool. Talk to your doctor about testing, especially if you have stomach pain or history of stomach ulcers. Once confirmed, there are several different protocols for treating *H. pylori* infection. Most include a proton pump inhibitor and one to two different antibiotic treatments for up to two weeks. In the world of integrative medicine, some practitioners wish to use natural herbal remedies like oregano, ginger, and thyme for eradication, with varying results. Either way, if you or a loved one is infected with *H. pylori*, getting rid of the bacteria is an important step in reducing autoimmunity and optimizing thyroid health.

■ Less Common Infections

In addition to the more common infections listed above, there are other infectious triggers that have been associated with the development of AITD. These include coxsackievirus, hepatitis C, Lyme disease, and diarrhea inducing bacteria like *Yersinia entercolitica* and *Blastocystis hominis*. For review, a full table of infectious triggers can be found in Chapter 3.

Although you have probably never heard of some of these, there is testing and treatment available for them, which is why it is important to work with your doctor to determine if there is an underlying infectious disease that maybe triggering or worsening thyroid autoimmunity. Treatment of underlying disease is important in calming inflammation and quieting the immune response; in turn, this can be key in improving symptoms of AITD.

COMMON DRUG EXPOSURES IN HASHIMOTO'S

Just like infectious disease exposures, certain over-the-counter and prescription drugs can also worsen autoimmunity. Here we will present some of the most common over-the-counter and prescription drugs that can worsen AITD. If you or a loved one is taking one of these medicines, it is worth discussing with your doctor if there are alternative options that might be better in your case.

■ Stomach Acid Reducers

If you walk down the medicine aisle at the drug store, you will likely see many options to treat indigestion. Several of these options are medicines called proton pump inhibitors (or PPIs). Common names include Prilosec Protonix, Nexium, Prevacid, and Aciphex. Because they are widely advertised and because acid indigestion is rampant in our society, many people take these to alleviate the pain.

But are they causing harm? Think back to our discussion on the microbiome and how maintaining good guy bacteria is so important in protecting the gut stonewall and calming fighting gut. In fact, one of the best ways to maintain the good guys is to make sure that any bad bacteria that you eat in your food are killed by your stomach acid!

Unfortunately, being on a long-term PPI reduces your stomach acid — which is exactly what it is supposed to do in order to reduce acid indigestion—and this unintentionally allows the bad guys to pass right down into the gut, triggering fighting gut and worsening AITD. Therefore, limiting exposure to PPIs is important in maintaining a healthy gut barrier and calming autoimmunity.

OUR ADVICE: Consider trying the following approaches to combating your acid reflux without the use of PPIs.

- Eliminate possible food triggers like dairy.

- Ensure that you do not have underlying H. pylori infection.

- Limit (or eliminate) caffeine, red wine, and spicy foods.

- Lose weight if needed. Excess weight can worsen acid reflux and indigestion.

- Try a more natural approach, such as using betaine HCl with pepsin or papaya enzyme extract to help with digestion of meals, or drinking eight ounces of water with one teaspoon of baking soda, apple cider vinegar, or ginger.

■ NSAIDs

Another overly used class of drugs that could be detrimental to your gut microbiome include nonsteroidal anti-inflammatory drugs, commonly referred to as NSAIDs. You might know them better by their commercial names which include Advil, Aleve, or Motrin. Studies have shown that taking NSAIDs daily over a long period of time is responsible for a marked reduction of lactobacilli, the most common good guy bacteria in the gut. Additionally, NSAIDs have been shown to reduce the health of the gut stonewall, contributing to development of fighting gut.

OUR ADVICE: If you can take Tylenol, it might be a better over-the-counter option for retaining a healthy microflora. More natural pain relievers include heat and cold, topical menthol, bromelain, evening primrose oil, ginger, turmeric, capsaicin, valerian root, cats claw, boswellia, CBD oil, and white willow bark.

Prescription Drugs

In addition to these detrimental over-the-counter options, there are certain prescription drugs that can negatively alter the microbiome or contribute to the development of autoimmunity. In Chapter 5, we presented a table of medications that can influence thyroid hormone metabolism. Some of these medications can also contribute directly to thyroid autoimmunity. In Table 11.1 are the most commonly prescribed medications that can contribute to or worsen Hashimoto's disease. If you are on any of these medications, you should consider discussing alternative options with your doctor, whenever possible.

In addition to avoiding the medications that contribute to AITD, limit your antibiotic use, and only take antibiotics when absolutely necessary and prescribed by your doctor. Taking antibiotics too often can make you sick by altering your microbiome and contributing to worsened autoimmunity. Still, it is sometimes necessary to take these prescription drugs to treat illness. In this situation, taking probiotics even during antibiotic therapy can help maintain a healthy gut barrier and optimize thyroid health.

TABLE 11.1. PRESCRIPTION MEDICINES THAT CAN WORSEN AUTOIMMUNE THYROID DISEASE	
PRESCRIPTION DRUG	**WHY IT WORSENS AITD**
Amiodarone (used for heart conditions)	Amiodarone has a lot of iodine in it, and too much iodine can worsen AITD
Antibiotics (excessive use)	Alters the gut microbiome and can worsen autoimmunity
Cancer Therapies (Ipilimumab, Lenvatinib, Nivolumab, Octreotide, Pembrolizumab, Sorafenib, Sunitinib, γ-Interferon, 5-FU)	Alters the immune system and can cause autoimmune disease
Estrogens and estrogen disruptors (including Clomid, Femara, Raloxifene, Tamoxifen)	Alters the gut microbiome and can worsen autoimmunity
Iodinated Contrast (Angiography and CT scans)	Too much iodine can worsen AITD

POLLUTANTS AND ALLERGENS

There are environmental toxins and synthetic man-made chemicals all around us. They are in the air we breathe, the water we drink, the food we eat, the cars we drive, and the household products we use. Alarmingly, many of these chemicals have never been tested in regard to human disease. We are well aware of environmental exposures, such as asbestos, which are strongly linked to forms of lung cancer. But did you know that inhalation of asbestos has also been shown to contribute to autoimmunity? In fact, there are many other chemicals in the environment associated with development of autoimmunity.

For example, living close to industrial air emissions is associated with an increased risk. Here's another example—years after the 9/11 attack in New York City, the emergency first responders at Ground Zero, having been exposed to multiple airborne chemicals, were found to have a significantly higher incidence of autoimmune disease, including rheumatoid arthritis and lupus. Similarly, lifelong exposure to chemicals in our environment increases the risk for AITD. But what are the most important environmental chemicals to avoid in Hashimoto's disease? Though research uncovers more about chemical exposures every day, currently, the chemicals most strongly linked to thyroid disease include:

- cigarette smoke
- phytoestrogens
- halogenated compounds
- radiation
- mercury and heavy metals

Despite the different categories of environmental exposures, all triggers likely work the same way. After being inhaled, absorbed through the skin, or ingested, these chemicals alter your body's normal protein structures to become new, foreign proteins, called "neoantigens." These neoantigens trigger your T and B cells to declare war and increase the autoimmune response. Once exposed, many of these chemicals accumulate within the body and are *never* excreted or removed. As we will see in the sections that follow, the best way to protect yourself is to reduce your lifetime exposure.

Thyroid Quick Tip: We are exposed to chemicals every single day. Many remain within the body for life because they are not easily removed. Therefore, to reduce Hashimoto's antibodies and prevent the development of autoimmune disease, it is important to reduce exposure to chemicals strongly linked to thyroid cancer and AITD.

■ Cigarette Smoke

By now we know that cigarette smoke is bad for health. It has been long associated with the development of lung cancer and cardiovascular disease. Interestingly, it has also been associated with the development of autoimmune disease. Cigarette smoke is inhaled through the lungs, which is another place in the body where T and B cell soldiers wait to check the identification of invaders in our bodies. Once inhaled, chemicals in cigarettes adhere to normal proteins in the body, forming neoantigens or "Frankenstein-like molecules" that are foreign to our immune cells. And what do they do when they see these foreign molecules? They attack!

There is a very strong association between cigarette smoking and Graves' disease. In fact, we know that cigarettes significantly increase TRAbs, the thyroid antibodies that contribute to hyperthyroidism. Smoking has also been shown to worsen the eye bulging often seen in those with Grave's disease. Even worse, smoking increases the risk for thyroid nodules and possibly even thyroid cancer. Cigarette smoking is also the most conclusively established risk factor for development of rheumatoid arthritis, lupus, and multiple sclerosis.

OUR ADVICE: Don't smoke. If you smoke, try to quit. There are options, which include nicotine replacement patches or gum, and smoking cessation prescriptions. Always talk to your doctor about whether or not these options are suitable for you. Everyone should reduce their exposure to secondhand smoke.

■ Mercury and Cadmium

If you were to look at the periodic table, you would see that there are several additional chemical elements in the same column as zinc, which, as we previously discussed, is one of the most important thyroid-specific vitamins. Two of these elements include mercury (Hg) and cadmium (Cd). Because of chemical similarities, both mercury and cadmium can displace zinc and contribute to development of thyroid disease.

Research shows that cadmium can increase risk for hypothyroidism. Interestingly, cadmium is also a big component of cigarette smoke. Cadmium is found in the Earth's crust, therefore we can be exposed to it from any product that's grown in the ground. Commercial products with the highest concentrations include batteries, QLED TVs, solar panels, and pigmented glass and plastics.

OUR ADVICE: If you can, avoid exposure to these high cadmium items. Alternatively, wash your hands after exposure and use non-pigmented glass and plastics.

With regard to mercury, studies have demonstrated that mercury toxicity can increase thyroglobulin antibodies (TgAbs), one of the most common antibodies in Hashimoto's disease. In fact, the National Health and Nutrition Examination Survey (NHANES), a very large and respected research group, did one of these studies, demonstrating that women who had higher mercury blood levels had twice the likelihood of having positive TgAbs. Additional studies have demonstrated that high exposure to mercury contributes to hypothyroidism. This begs the question—what are our biggest exposures to mercury?

We are most often exposed to mercury in fish and in dental fillings (also called amalgams). Because we know the source of our biggest exposures, there are some things that we can do to reduce our total body burden of mercury. In addition, unlike some of the other chemicals discussed in this chapter, mercury levels can be reduced by medications (in a process called chelation). Work with your doctor to determine if testing your blood mercury levels is important.

OUR ADVICE: Eat lower mercury fish. In Table 11.2 on page 162, we have listed many types of fish and their typical mercury content. Remember that mercury concentration depends on where the fish was raised and its lifetime exposure to mercury—information that is almost impossible to obtain. Do your best to reduce mercury exposure by choosing fish typically low in mercury.

There are a few additional measures you can take to further reduce your exposure to mercury.

Choose mercury-free dental fillings, or consider replacement of mercury-laden fillings. It is worth noting that, although The American Dental Association maintains that mercury fillings are safe, they are rarely used anymore. However, many older fillings do contain mercury. Not everyone with mercury fillings needs to have them removed. In fact, some studies show no association between mercury fillings and Hashimoto's disease. Still, if you have multiple mercury fillings and very high Tg antibodies, it

TABLE 11.2. MERCURY CONCENTRATIONS IN FISH		
LOW MERCURY FISH TO ENJOY	**MODERATE MERCURY FISH TO EAT IN MODERATION (6 SERVINGS OR LESS/MONTH)**	**HIGH MERCURY FISH TO AVOID**
Atlantic mackerel	Black bass	Ahi tuna
Butterfish	Canned light tuna	Albacore tuna
Catfish	Cod	Bigeye tuna
Chub mackerel	Freshwater perch	Blue fish
Clam	Halibut	Grouper
Crab	Lobster	Gulf mackerel
Crawfish	Mahi-mahi	King mackerel
Croaker	Salt water bath	Marlin
Flounder	Sea trout	Orange roughy
Freshwater trout	Skipjack tuna	Sea bass
Haddock	Striped bass	Shark
Herring	Trout	Spanish mackerel
Mullet	White fish	Swordfish
Muscles		Tilefish
Oysters		Yellowfin tuna
Perch		
Pollock		
Rainbow trout		
Salmon		
Sardines		
Scallops		
Shrimp		
Sole		
Squid		
Tilapia		

may be reasonable to consider removal. There are dentists that specialize in doing this, called biological dentists. Head to our resources section to learn how to find one near you.

Avoid multi-dose vaccines. Although most vaccines nowadays no longer contain a form of mercury called thimerosal, several vaccines still contain small amounts. These include DT (diphtheria and tetanus), TD (tetanus and diphtheria), and TT (tetanus toxoid). Still, thimerosal can still be found in adult multi-dose vaccines (meaning vials that contain multiple doses of the vaccine used for multiple patients), particularly the flu shot. Fluvirin and Fluzone are names of the multidose forms. When you find yourself required to take these vaccines, make sure you ask for a single dose vaccine vial that doesn't contain thimerosal.

If you get a tattoo, avoid red ink. Although tattoos have become more popular over the years, they are not completely risk-free when it comes to disrupting the immune system. Most red inks used to create tattoos contain mercury and can contain other harmful heavy metals, including cadmium. Other tattoo colors can contain toxic heavy metals, including arsenic and lead, that can contribute to other forms of human disease. So if you're getting a tattoo, choose black ink. Alternatively, you can look for more eco-friendly, non-metallic ink alternatives.

■ Radiation

Exposure to radiation is the best-known risk factor for development of thyroid cancer. Some of the most common radiation exposures include multiple x-rays without a thyroid shield, particularly in early childhood, and external beam radiation used as part of cancer treatment. In addition to healthcare-related radiation exposures like x-rays, CT scans, and radiation treatments for cancer, there are multiple radioactive elements that are found naturally in the Earth's crust. Humans are exposed to these elements as they rise to the Earth's surface and accumulate in crops, animals, water, and air.

In fact, it has been shown that people living near volcanoes are exposed to more of these radioactive elements (specifically, naturally occurring radium and thallium) and have an increased risk for thyroid cancer. Naturally occurring radon in basements, on the other hand, has not been definitively linked to thyroid disease. It has also been theorized, but not proven, that pilots and flight attendants may also be at risk for increased atmospheric radiation, thereby contributing to development of thyroid cancer. Additionally, nuclear power plant explosions and nuclear bombs are well-established risk factors for thyroid cancer.

■ Phytoestrogens

Phytoestrogens are plant-derived estrogen-like compounds found in food, cosmetic products, lotions, and even some essential oils. These estrogen-like products primarily work to alter thyroid function by increasing or decreasing the proteins that bind thyroid hormone. In large amounts, they can significantly worsen hypothyroidism.

In food sources, the most common phytoestrogens are soy and stilbenes, namely phytoestrogens found in red grapes and wine. As we discussed in Chapter 9, ingestion of these items in moderation is perfectly fine for most Hashimoto's patients, but excess exposure may worsen thyroid issues.

Nuclear Power Plants and Thyroid Effects

You might be surprised to know that people living near a nuclear power plant do not generally have higher rates of thyroid cancer. Though still being studied, research suggests that close proximity alone does not cause thyroid cancer, although living near a nuclear power plant *has* been associated with other health issues, like breathing problems from air emissions.

However, when there is a nuclear power disaster, meltdown, or explosion, the release of radiation is correlated with higher rates of thyroid cancer, as well as higher thyroid antibody levels. When there is a nuclear disaster, radioactive iodine is released into the environment. The thyroid absorbs radioactive iodine, just like it does regular iodine. Because of this, it is recommended that people living close to nuclear power plants take precautions. If you live within 10 miles of a nuclear power plant, you should make sure to get potassium iodide (also called KI) pills from participating local government or health offices.

Pills are taken before or up to three hours after exposure to radioactive iodine. One dose of 130 mg protects the thyroid for twenty-four hours. In theory, it gives you enough time to evacuate a dangerous situation. The government will notify residents if there is an event that necessitates taking the pill. People should not take potassium iodide unless they are told to do so, as it can have side effects.

After taking potassium iodide, the pill works by flooding the thyroid with a form of stable iodide, which blocks the absorption of any radioactive iodine. It only protects the thyroid from radiation, not any other parts of the body. Although the thyroid absorbs more iodine—radioactive or not—than other areas of the body, some is absorbed in the bone marrow and the gut.

If you do live near a radioactive facility of any type, a bottle of potassium iodide should be kept on-hand. Potassium iodide can be purchased online, without a prescription.

Anti-aging cosmetic products and skin creams can also contain phytoestrogens; look for and avoid resveratrol, equol, or genistein in the label. If your thyroid levels are difficult to control, electing for antiaging skin care products that are low in phytoestrogens may be beneficial.

Parabens are another example of phytoestrogens commonly found in cosmetic products, lotions, and perfumes. Like many of the chemicals in our cosmetics, we are exposed to them through absorption in the skin. They have been shown in multiple studies to influence thyroid hormone metabolism. Avoid products with parabens listed among the ingredients. Common parabens include: methylparaben, propylparaben, butylparaben, and heptylparaben.

Certain essential oils also act as phytoestrogens and can impact the protein that binds to thyroid hormone, thereby altering thyroid hormone concentration of blood. The worst offenders? Lavender and tea tree oil. Most other essential oils do not act as phytoestrogens.

When estrogen-like products are artificially manufactured, they are also sometimes referred to as *xenoestrogens*. Xenoestrogens, like bisphenol A (BPA) and phthalates, are commonly found in plastics and used as a lining in most food and beverage containers. There is abundant data demonstrating that BPA and certain phthalates do, in fact, adversely affect thyroid hormone levels in multiple populations. Serum BPA has also been associated with increased TPOAbs, the most common Hashimoto's antibody.

TABLE 11.3. COMMON PRODUCTS WITH PHYTOESTROGENS	
TYPE OF PHYTOESTROGEN	COMMON PRODUCTS
BPA/Phthalates	Baby bottles, canned food (BPA found in the can liner), food storage plastic containers, hair care products, IV bags and tubing, medications (labeled time release or safety coated), nail polish, vinyl shower curtains, and plastic water bottles/sports drink bottles.
Essential oils	Air fresheners, body lotion, candles, perfumes, and supplements.
Parabens	Hair care products, moisturizer, makeup, and shaving products.

OUR ADVICE: Look for cosmetics, lotions, perfumes, and essential oils that are low in phytoestrogens. When buying plastics, look for BPA-free on the label, or even better, use glass containers.

■ Halogenated Compounds

Perhaps the most common and most frequent environmental exposure contributing to AITD are halogenated compounds. In Chapter 9, we discussed how dietary halogens, including brominated chemicals, fluoride, and sodium chloride, can disrupt iodide uptake by the thyroid gland and contribute to hypothyroidism. Unfortunately, halogenated compounds are not limited to our foods. They are everywhere, disguised as chemicals with long names in our cleaning supplies, household items, mattresses, couch covers, and electronic equipment.

Most often, polybrominated (meaning many bromides) diphenyl ethers (PBDEs), and polychlorinated biphenyls (PCBs) are cited as common thyroid disruptors. Additionally, fluorinated compounds like per- and polyfluoroalkyl substances (PFAS), a group of man-made chemicals that include PFOA, PFOS, and GenX, are associated with thyroid disruption. The next time you're at the hardware store or in the cleaning aisle at the grocery store, *read the list of ingredients.* You will be surprised to see how many chemical names have different forms of bromide, chloride, and fluoride on the label.

Many of these brominated and chlorinated compounds, including PBDEs and PCBs, are also flame-retardants and found in many household electronics, vehicles, mattresses, and couches. To meet the fire safety standards, fire resistant chemicals are added to products to slow or prevent fires. In fact, the *Chicago Tribune* reported that a large couch contains up to two pounds of toxic flame retardant chemicals in its cushions.

Over time, these chemicals can leach out of the product into house dust that is then inhaled or ingested on unwashed hands, leading to chronic human exposure. Many of these PCBE chemicals look like thyroid hormone to the body. Thus, chronic exposure has been shown to be associated with both hypothyroidism and hyperthyroidism. In addition, several PCBEs have also been associated with increased risk for papillary thyroid cancer.

So where are our most common household exposures to these chemicals? We have listed them in the following table. Keep in mind that most halogenated products are reasonably safe when used minimally or in moderation, and the level of toxicity is dependent on how often the product is used and the length of exposure.

OUR ADVICE: If practical, look for substitute products that are not brominated, chlorinated, or fluorinated and, if no substitute is available, limit exposure. Alternatively, you can make your own cleaning solutions from more natural items like white vinegar, castile soap, baking soda, and lemons. Head to our resource section for more suggestions on where to buy nontoxic household products.

TABLE 11.4. COMMON HOUSEHOLD CHEMICALS	
CHEMICAL NAME	**PRODUCTS**
Brominated Compounds	**Found in the Following Products**
HBCDs, PBDEs, PCBs, and TBBPAs	• Auto upholstery and car electronics • Carpet padding • Electronic equipment (cell phones, computers, fax machines, remote control products, stereos, wires, and TVs) • Furniture (foam) • Gym mats (foam) • Household insulation • Imitation wood • Mattresses (foam) • Paints • Plastics
Potassium bromide	• Photo supplies/developer
Chlorinated Compounds	**Found in the Following Products**
Alkyl ammonium chlorides	• Eye drops • Pool chemicals
Chlorinated tris flame retardant	• Children's pajamas • Foam-containing baby products
Chlorpyrifos	• Bug spray and pesticides
Calcium hypochlorite, hydrochloric acid, sodium hypochlorite	• Bleach • Cleaning products • Mold and mildew removers • Pool chemicals • Toilet bowl cleaners
Perchlorates and perchloroethylene (PERC)	• Dry cleaning • Rug, carpet, upholstery cleaners • Water and food contamination (specifically cow's milk)
P-dichlorobenzene (p-DCB)	• Air fresheners • Mold and mildew removers • Mothballs • Urinal deodorizer

Fluorinated Compounds	Found in the Following Products
Dichlorodifluoromethane	• Freon-12 (auto supply, air conditioner)
PFAS (PFOA/PFOS/GenX)	• Cleaning products
	• Contaminated drinking water (from firefighter foams water and soil close to airports and military bases)
	• Nonstick products (Teflon products, including popcorn bags and pizza boxes)
	• Nonstick cookware
	• Paints
	• Polishes
	• Stain and water repellent fabrics
	• Waxes

Reducing your exposure to these chemicals is the most important intervention that you can make. Once exposed, these chemicals remain in the body and are impossible to remove. Therefore, we sometimes refer to environmental exposures in Hashimoto's as "total toxic load," referring to all cumulative chemical exposures. As one gets older, the total toxic load increases due to increasing years of chemical exposure. Your goal? To minimize these thyroid-specific chemical exposures and reduce your total toxic load as you age.

Thyroid Quick Tip: As a general rule of thumb, avoid or use protection when working with cleaning products, paints, polishes, and other products with bromide, chloride, and fluoride (or any forms of these words with chemical names, such as bromo/chloro/fluoro) in the label. Protection includes goggles, gloves, and a facemask. As you can see, it is near impossible to avoid flame-retardants in electronics and furniture, but maintaining minimal house dust where it accumulates and washing your hands before eating to remove chemicals is helpful.

As discussed, there are ways to protect yourself from these toxic chemicals, but sometimes exposure is unavoidable. When brominated and chlorinated flame retardants burn, they give off extremely toxic brominated, chlorinated, and bromo-chlorinated dioxins and furans as fumes. These chemicals are then released into the atmosphere, contaminating human food sources, water, and have even been found in human breast milk. In

Five Easy Steps
to Reduce Your Total Toxic Load

The greater your toxic load, the more disruptions to your immune system. You can reduce your overall toxic load by following these simple steps.

1. Buy products without halogenated chemicals, if possible, and elect for home furnishings that don't require the addition of flame-retardants. These materials include aramide blend (Kevlar), glass, hemp, leather, metal, pre-ceramic polymers, and wool.

2. Minimize house dust.

3. Change your household air filters regularly.

4. Wash your hands prior to eating or touching your mouth.

5. When using these toxic chemicals, wear gloves (Viton gloves), goggles, or a facemask to reduce your exposure.

fact, there are reports that these chemical substances have been detected in polar bears living in the uninhabited parts of the Arctic Circle. Therefore, do your best to avoid excess exposure in your everyday life, but know, unfortunately, that these chemicals are everywhere in our environment. As we raise awareness that these chemicals can contribute to thyroid disorders and human disease, we can hope that changes will be made to decrease toxic chemical exposures for future generations.

CONCLUSION

We now know that there are a variety of environmental exposures that affect Hashimoto's, including infections, drugs, allergens, and pollutants. Although it is impossible to avoid everything in the environment that can cause negative effects in AITD, you can reduce your exposure by following the suggestions we have discussed in this chapter. Next, we will explore the ways in which you can optimize thyroid levels and reduce Hashimoto's flares.

12.

Reducing Hashimoto's Flares and Optimizing Thyroid Levels

Throughout the book, we have discussed many aspects of Hashimoto's Disease, ranging from the different thyroid medications to dietary strategies and environmental factors that may influence overall thyroid health. In this chapter, we will discuss effective practical tips and tricks that you can use to reduce Hashimoto's flares and optimize your thyroid health. But first, what do we mean by "Hashimoto's flares"?

HASHIMOTO'S FLARES

Just like you can have a flare-up of any other autoimmune disease, such as rheumatoid arthritis or multiple sclerosis, you can also have a flare-up of AITD. A Hashimoto's flare normally occurs over a short period of time, usually one to two weeks, when Hashimoto's symptoms get noticeably worse. Moving forward on your thyroid journey, it is important to know how to recognize Hashimoto's flares and develop strategies to avoid them.

How to Recognize a Hashimoto's Flare

As we discussed in Chapter 3, there are multiple forms of Hashimoto's thyroiditis associated with a range of symptoms that may differ from patient to patient. Some patients with Hashimoto's disease have tenderness along the front of their neck; others have a pulling sensation at the base of the neck that sometimes makes it difficult to swallow; still others don't have any neck symptoms, but have times in their thyroid journey when they just feel "off." All of these symptoms can be exacerbated during a flare.

Symptoms of a Hashimoto's flare can be dramatically different between patients and can change within the same patient over time. Some patients have worsening neck tenderness, while others experience worsening fatigue and Hashimoto's symptoms. Some patients experience multiple flares many times a year, while others never experience a flare at all. This begs the question—why do Hashimoto's flares happen?

Flare-Up Symptoms

While symptoms might be familiar to your day-to-day Hashimoto's symptoms, some may not. Here are the most common symptoms likely to be present during a flare:

- anxiety or depression
- brain fog
- flu-like symptoms without the flu
- general worsening feeling of weakness or malaise
- neck pain, pressure, or swelling

- sleeping more than usual or more difficulty getting out of bed
- sudden onset of worsened hypo *or* hyper thyroid symptoms
- worsening of fatigue
- increased muscle or joint pain

Why Do Flares Happen?

Many times Hashimoto's flares begin after exposure to a trigger. Some of these triggers include:

- food, medication, or environmental allergies
- sleep deprivation

- stress
- viral, bacterial, or fungal infections

Thyroid Quick Tip: It is important to recognize and understand a typical flare symptom pattern, so you can recognize it if and when it happens. If you have increased neck tenderness, pain, or worsened Hashimoto's symptoms that last more than a few days, you're probably in a flare. If it's the first time you've felt your AITD flaring up, contact your doctor. If you've had flares before, but are experiencing one that is prolonged or severe, contact your doctor.

What do all of these triggers have in common? They all stimulate an immune response! And as we have found out in previous chapters, triggering the already confused immune system in AITD can worsen its attack on the thyroid gland. These times of increased immune attacks on the thyroid gland constitute Hashimoto's flares. Whether patients have flares and how often they have them vary. Why would this be?

The best explanation is that flares may occur more commonly in patients who developed AITD due to a viral trigger. Conversely, patients who developed AITD after a bacterial, fungal, allergic, or stressful immune trigger may not have as many flares, particularly if the triggering event has been definitively treated or is now being avoided. The exception to this is patients who are continuously exposed to a food or environmental allergen that may be continuously triggering their immune response. In that case, avoidance of these triggers is of utmost importance in reducing flare-ups.

The Unique Role of Viruses and Hashimoto's Flares

So why do patients with viral triggers have an increased risk for Hashimoto's flares? As previously mentioned, viral infections including EBV and HHV-6 are among the most common triggers for AITD. They are the most common triggers because viral particles are *everywhere*. In fact, there are so many different viruses that, if we were to stack viruses one on top of each other, they would reach 100 million light years into space. In fact, because we are all continuously exposed to viruses throughout our life, humans have co-evolved with viruses over the past 400 million years. In fact, some reports suggest that up to 42 percent of the human genome is comprised of viral sequences. Isn't that crazy?

Most of the time, the viruses within us are latent, meaning that they hang out inactive and unrecognized within our cells, living in harmony with our immune system. Think of this relationship as some sort of peace treaty where we allow them to hang out if they stay quiet. Under stress, illness, or after exposure to allergens, however, they can rear their ugly heads and reactivate.

Let's look at an example. You or someone you know may get fever blisters or cold sores, typically after a severe cold or after a stressful life event. Cold sores are one example of a latent herpes virus reactivating during times of host illness or stress. Other examples of viruses that reactivate after times of stress or infection include shingles and latent chickenpox, another herpes virus. Because the Epstein-Barr virus (EBV) and

Human Herpesvirus 6 (HHV-6) are also both members of the herpes family, stressful triggers or infection can similarly reactivate the viruses and cause an ugly immune response, leading to a Hashimoto's flare. Be aware that the herpes viruses associated with AITD are not sexually transmitted diseases (STDs). There are nine herpes associated viruses that commonly infect humans, most of which are not considered STDs.

Whenever you get an infection or are stressed, for example, your T and B cells send out signals throughout the body, alerting it to the fact that it is under attack. These signals help to recruit other immune cells to effectively fight the infection or stressor. Unbeknownst to your T and B cells, the signals also notify your latent viral infections that the body they are living in is under attack. And these viral infections aren't stupid—they aren't going to hang around in an unhealthy host who is stressed and sick!

Instead of sticking around, they reactivate in a valiant attempt to infect another healthy person, thereby protecting and preserving the virus for future generations. Because of this process, AITD patients with latent viral infections tend to get more severe flares after triggering events. In fact, there have been studies where a fine needle biopsy of the Hashimoto's thyroid gland uncovered EBV virus hiding within the thyroid cells, supporting the reactivation concept.

Now that we have a better idea of how flares occur, we will discuss some strategies to reduce or avoid them altogether.

REDUCING HASHIMOTO'S FLARES

There are several strategies that can be used to reduce or avoid Hashimoto's flares. Remember, everyone is different and some strategies may work for one person while others may have flares regardless of what they do. Additionally, over time an individual's triggers may change, necessitating reevaluation and an altered game plan. Nevertheless, here are three easy steps to reducing Hashimoto's flares:

■ Step 1: Identify Your Triggers

Many times, Hashimoto's flares occur days to weeks after exposure to an inciting trigger, making it difficult to pinpoint the triggering event. Other times, patients have flares without ever knowing what caused them. Keeping a journal of symptoms, stress level, and foods may be helpful to keep around the time of a flare to identify any potential environmental triggers and work to avoid them in the future. Washing one's hands and reducing exposure to additional viral and bacterial infections is also important in quieting the immune response. Table 12.1 will provide you with an example of how you can set up a journal or log to document and recognize your triggers.

TABLE 12.1. HASHIMOTO'S TRIGGERS LOG					
DATE	FOODS EATEN	STRESS (LOW, MEDIUM, HIGH)	SLEEP (QUANTITY & QUALITY)	ALLERGIES OR ILLNESS (Y OR N)	SYMPTOMS

Symptoms may or may not be related to a flare. After journaling for several months, it may be helpful to go back through the information and identify daily symptoms versus occasional symptoms that seem to come and go. While daily symptoms must be treated, they are more likely coming from Hashimoto's itself. The occasional symptoms, on the other hand, are more likely to constitute a Hashimoto's flare.

Once identified, look back at the foods, stress level, sleep quality, and allergies or illness you experience on the day symptoms appear and for one to two weeks prior. Many times, patients will be able to identify a common trigger or triggers. If you are lucky enough to identify a trigger, do your best to avoid it in the upcoming months and reevaluate whether the frequency of your flares has improved. It is important to keep a log of symptoms throughout your Hashimoto's journey, as symptoms and triggers may change with time.

■ Step 2: Reduce Your AITD Antibodies

Quieting the immune response and reducing Hashimoto's flares is desirable, but is it possible to go into full remission? In some patients, yes! The ability for AITD patients to go into remission depends on the inciting immune trigger, the severity of the autoimmune response, and how well the patient can calm his or her immune response by avoiding triggers. Patients who have had bacterial, fungal, allergic or stressful AITD triggers are much more likely to be able to go into full remission, meaning a complete reduction in antibodies and symptoms. Those who have had a mild viral infection and immune response are also good candidates for remission.

In fact, the literature suggest that up to 30 percent of patients with Graves' disease (and in Dr. Henderson's experience, closer to 60 percent) can get into full remission, whereas the likelihood of remission in Hashimoto's disease really depends on the inciting trigger, length of disease (the earlier it is caught, the better), and the severity of the individual's immune response. For example, Hashimoto's patients who have had a severe viral trigger, high residual viral load, and a prolonged immune response do not often go into remission completely.

Conversely, Hashimoto's patients who are early in their thyroid journey, are diligently avoiding triggers, have lower antibody titers, have never had a viral trigger, or have a low residual viral load if they did have a viral trigger, tend to go into remission more easily. Specific patient groups, including those with longstanding Hashimoto's disease, Hashitoxicosis, and severe Graves' disease (with very high antibody titers), are much less likely to go into remission. The ability to go into remission from AITD depends on multiple factors, which are listed in Table 12.2.

TABLE 12.2. AITD REMISSION	
LESS LIKELY TO ACHIEVE REMISSION	**MORE LIKELY TO ACHIEVE REMISSION**
Chronic infection	Bacterial, fungal, environmental or stressful triggers that have been treated
Hashitoxicosis	
High antibodies	Early AITD
High residual viral load	Lower antibody titers
Longstanding Hashimoto's disease (more than 10 years)	Patient diligently avoids triggers
Severe Graves' disease (high Abs)	Viral triggers with a lower residual viral load
Patient is not avoiding triggers	

Even if you find yourself in the "less likely to achieve remission" box, you can still make a dramatic impact on your disease state. In these cases, reduction of AITD antibodies is of utmost importance in quieting immune symptoms. In addition to limiting triggers and exposures, there are several effective ways to lower AITD antibodies.

4 Steps to Reducing AITD Antibodies

- Avoid Your Triggers
- Thyroid Replacement
- Improve the Immune System
- Decrease Inflammation

Avoid Your Triggers

Once identified, the most important way to reduce AITD antibodies is to avoid known triggers. If you are gluten sensitive or have celiac disease, for example, eliminating gluten from your diet may dramatically improve your antibodies. If you have a chronic environmental allergy exposure such as pet dander or house dust, investing in an air purifying system, replacing carpets, and reducing daily exposures to allergens can quiet the immune response and positively impact AITD. If you smoke, there is good data to support that stopping will help reduce your AITD antibodies, particularly in Graves' disease.

Reducing viral infections and treating underlying bacterial infections is also important in decreasing thyroid antibodies. In addition, studies have demonstrated that patients with high levels of mercury and iodine exposure have higher levels of TgAbs. Therefore, limiting food and environmental exposures is the first step in reducing AITD antibodies.

Improve the Immune System

As discussed in Chapter 9, improving diet to reducing fighting gut dramatically improves the T and B cell soldier response to immune triggers. Additionally, in Chapter 10, we discussed how various supplements help bolster the immune response. For example, most studies suggest that the addition of selenium at doses up 200 to 400 mcg daily decreases both TPOAbs and TRAbs by 40 percent.

In addition, studies have demonstrated that patients with high levels of mercury and iodine exposure have higher levels of TgAbs. Therefore, reducing environmental exposures and excess iodine is important in improving the immune response. A final way to impact the immune system is with immunomodulators, or natural or prescription medications that have significant effects on quieting the immune response. In previous chapters, we mentioned several of these, including black cumin oil and low-dose naltrexone (LDN), two treatments that have some supporting evidence for AITD antibody reduction in specific individuals.

Berberine and curcumin are additional supplements that have been shown to quiet immunity. Prescription immunomodulator therapies like methotrexate, cyclosporine, and many of the monoclonal antibodies (any drug that is difficult to pronounce and ends with "mab"), like rituximab, do not have good data for reducing antibodies in AITD, but are shown to have some efficacy in Graves' eye disease. These are extremely serious medications, and any consideration for prescription immunomodulator therapy should be discussed in detail with your doctor.

Thyroid Replacement

One of the strongest factors in reducing AITD antibodies is normalizing the TSH. When TSH is high, AITD antibodies like TPO and Tg also increase. The simple step of starting thyroid replacement medicine and optimizing TSH into the normal range can decrease antibodies by up to an astonishing 50 to 60 percent! In fact, there have been studies that demonstrate that simply going on levothyroxine thyroid replacement medicine for at least three years can put many Hashimoto's patients with TBII, a special type of blocking antibody, into remission and allow them to come off thyroid medicine completely.

With regard to more natural thyroid replacement options, there is some thought that taking natural products like Armour and Nature-throid can actually increase AITD antibodies. This is because the desiccated pig thyroid gland contains pig Tg and TPO proteins that can *theoretically* increase and cross-react with the human AITD antibodies. Clinically, though, we do not see that natural replacement options worsen AITD antibodies, and there are no studies to support this. If there is clinical concern, checking AITD antibodies three months after starting desiccated porcine thyroid replacement is reasonable. Overall, starting on thyroid replacement medicine, even for a short time, can significantly reduce your antibody load.

Decrease Inflammation

Reducing whole body inflammation is key to decreasing AITD antibodies. For example, there is data to show that high-dose statin therapy can dramatically reduce Hashimoto's antibodies. How can this be? Although statins are typically used to lower high cholesterol, they also have anti-inflammatory and immunomodulary properties.

In a lipid study, changes in AITD antibodies directly correlated with a decrease in C-reactive protein (CRP), a marker of inflammation. Therefore, reducing inflammation is of utmost importance in quieting the immune response. Inflammation can result from multiple disease processes including osteoarthritis, fibromyalgia, asthma, chronic dental infections, or fighting gut. Treating inflammatory diseases can have a positive response on systemic inflammation, thereby reducing AITD antibodies. Reducing exposure to inflammatory foods, like artificial ingredients and sugar, is also important. Lastly, taking anti-inflammatory supplements as discussed in Chapter 10 is another key part in lowering AITD antibodies and improving symptoms.

Remember That This Is a Journey

Even if you were able to get your antibodies to come down significantly or disappear, triggers down the road could reinitiate a relapse and increase your antibodies and AITD symptoms once again. Therefore, we tend to think of AITD as a journey. There are times where patients can go into remission and times where symptoms can worsen. Reducing triggers, following a thyroid-specific diet and nutrition plan, and working to reduce your antibody load are of utmost importance in maintaining your thyroid health. Still, there is one final component to reducing Hashimoto's flares that is difficult for all of us—reducing *stress*.

■ Step 3: Reduce Your Stress!

One of the most important steps in reducing Hashimoto's flares is stress reduction. When doctors tell their patients that they need to reduce stress, most just laugh—and we totally get it! In today's society, we are bombarded with endless financial, social, and work-related stressors. Did you know that when your body is stressed, it sends out distress signals that dramatically affect your immune system? In fact, there is even data that maternal stress during pregnancy impacts immune system development of the fetus, potentially contributing to the development of allergies and autoimmunity in the offspring.

The body's reaction to stress is sometimes referred to as the "flight or fight response." In response to stress, an important part of the brain called the hypothalamus signals to the pituitary gland that the body is under attack and needs to either "fight back" or "take flight" by leaving the stressful situation. As part of the stress response, the pituitary gland stimulates the adrenal glands to produce stress hormones like adrenaline and cortisol. These hormones have many effects throughout the body. For example, they increase alertness and vigilance, focus attention, and increase the pain threshold in response to potential threats. But did you know that the stress response also has effects on the immune system?

Stress can affect the immune system in a variety of ways and is highly influenced by the *duration* of the stressor. Acute stressors can activate the immune response, whereas longstanding, chronic stress can decrease the immune response and increase the likelihood of disease and illness. Acute stressors, particularly during times when the host is already fighting illness, can increase the T and B cell response, recruiting untrained soldiers and thereby contribute to autoimmunity. Chronic stress is also a contributor to autoimmunity, though the mechanism is more complex and outside the scope of this book.

With regard to AITD, there have been multiple studies that link worsened autoimmune thyroid disease with stress, whereas others have been negative or inconclusive. Still, the literature is clear that stress negatively affects the immune response.

OUR ADVICE: Reducing stress needs to be a major priority in your thyroid journey.

Optimizing the Adrenals to Reduce Hashimoto's Flares

Many patients with AITD ask about "adrenal fatigue" as a contributor to fatigue and other symptoms. In fact, many sources suggest that a majority of AITD patients also have adrenal fatigue. But is adrenal fatigue a real thing? The term *adrenal fatigue* refers to an abnormal hypothalamic, pituitary, and adrenal (HPA) signaling response to stress.

Much like subclinical hypothyroidism, alternative medicine practitioners have labeled subclinical hypoadrenalism, or a less-than-robust HPA stress signaling response, as "adrenal fatigue." This is a diagnosis

Stress Reduction Ideas

Stress can and does make almost any illness worse, and as we have mentioned, this strongly applies to AITD flare-ups. We can't stress enough (pun intended) how big a role stress plays in Hashimoto's (and Graves') flare-ups. While definitely easier said than done, the more effective your efforts are in reducing stress, the more impact it will have on reducing flare-ups. These are some ways to reduce stress:

- **Practice Deep Breathing.** When we get stressed, we sometimes forget to breathe normally. Take a deep breath from your core—and let it out. Do this ten times.

- **Exercise Within Your Limits.** Even ten or fifteen minutes of light exercise can be helpful. Try to push yourself if you're having a hard time getting motivated, but *don't* push yourself to go beyond your physical limits.

- **Meditate.** Meditation is one of the most effective stress reducers. There are free apps and many websites that can teach you about meditation.

- **Listen to Music.** Turn up your favorite music and let yourself get absorbed in it. If you feel like dancing, even better.

- **Experience Nature.** Enjoy your morning coffee outside, go on a hike (that matches your energy level), or do some gardening.

- **Pray.** If you are a person of faith and this is something you feel comfortable doing, turn your stress over to a higher power.

- **Walk.** Just getting your body moving can help to stimulate stress-fighting hormones.

- **Write.** If you are stressed, try writing about it. Don't worry about what words you use, just write whatever thoughts or feelings come to mind. Get it out of your mind and body, and onto the page.

that is not currently recognized by mainstream medicine. Like anything else in medicine and science, that doesn't necessarily mean that the adrenal fatigue is a made-up thing, just like it turned out that the Earth wasn't flat after all! It does mean, however, that it has yet to be proven. Many patients will take adrenal support vitamins or steroids to support the adrenal system. In our opinion, there are several considerations with this approach.

Re-evaluate the Use of Glandulars

Many adrenal support vitamins contain desiccated porcine or bovine adrenal gland. Some contain pituitary gland. Glandulars refer to raw animal glands that are normally dried and grounded. Like other glandular products, it is important to know the source of the supplement, as poorly prepared glandular products can transmit disease. The best glandulars usually come from organic cows raised in New Zealand (where there have been no reports of mad cow disease) or organic fed cows raised on grass and without the use of pesticides, hormones, or antibiotics.

Still, there is no strong scientific data that supports their use in clinical practice. Additionally, the concentration of adrenal hormones like adrenaline is not FDA-regulated and can contribute to side effects like heart racing, high blood pressure, and headache.

OUR ADVICE: You may way to reconsider use of adrenal glandulars and, if you do elect to use them, work with a trained professional on choosing a safe option.

Know the Ingredients in Your Adrenal Support Supplements.

Adrenal support supplements also often contain licorice root or *Glycyrrhiza glabra*. In high concentrations, this ingredient can contribute to development of Cushing's Syndrome, or excess cortisol in the body. Side effects include weight gain, acne, hair growth on the face and chest, and stretch marks on the thighs and abdomen. Buyer beware!

OUR ADVICE: Consider avoiding supplements with licorice root on the label.

Avoid Unnecessary Steroids

Lastly, steroids like hydrocortisone, Cortef, or Prednisone are sometimes prescribed to help support the adrenal response. In actuality, taking these steroids confuses HPA axis signaling even more. They are unnecessary unless someone has a true diagnosis of adrenal insufficiency, or complete absence of adrenal response.

Adding steroids unnecessarily can also cause Cushing's syndrome, contribute to weight gain, weaken bones, and even worsen fatigue and muscle weakness. Additionally, steroid inhalers, creams, and injections used to treat asthma, COPD, arthritis, and skin conditions can also contribute to abnormal HPA axis signaling.

OUR ADVICE: Avoid steroids unless you have proven adrenal insufficiency (not just adrenal fatigue), or need them for another concurrent illness.

Tips to Support the Adrenals

So how can one support the adrenal response without causing further harm? Patients need to be aware that chronic stress, steroid and pain medications, and other illnesses, particularly sleep apnea and insomnia, can contribute to alterations in HPA axis signaling, thereby contributing to fatigue and worsened autoimmunity. Therefore, reducing stress, treating underlying illnesses, minimizing interfering medications, and optimizing nutrition that supports these stress-signaling pathways is of utmost importance in treating "adrenal fatigue."

Eat right, take recommended supplements, sleep well, and reduce stress, and you are well on your way to optimizing adrenal health and the stress response. The best supplements needed to support HPA signaling and adrenal function include vitamin C, vitamin B_1, vitamin B_5, vitamin B_6, vitamin B_{12}, and magnesium. Refer to Chapter 10 for dosages of vitamin C, vitamin B_1, and magnesium. Refer to Table 12.3 on the following page for the RDAs for vitamin B_5, B_6, and B_{12}.

Always discuss your vitamins and supplements with your doctor. Most multivitamins will contain B vitamins, but adding a B-complex vitamin might also be helpful. Even though taking vitamins can be helpful, eliminating stress, treating sleep apnea, and correcting insomnia are the most effective ways to improve HPA signaling.

OUR ADVICE: Reduce stress and work on effective, restful sleep to improve your HPA stress-signaling axis.

Optimizing the Gut to Reduce Hashimoto's Flares

In Chapter 9 and 10, we discussed proper nutrition and supplements to optimize the microbiome and improve fighting gut. In this chapter, we discussed stress reduction as an integral part of reducing AITD flares and improving symptoms. But did you know that gut health and health of the microbiome is intimately linked to the stress response? In fact, studies have demonstrated that bad guys in the gut microbiome can feed on chemicals like serotonin, gamma-aminobutyric acid (GABA), dopamine, and glutamate.

As a result, imbalances in these chemical messengers traveling to the brain can contribute to anxiety disorders, panic attacks, and worsened stress response. An unhealthy gut microbiome can result in too little serotonin, too much glutamate, and too little GABA, contributing to worsened anxiety. Therefore, optimizing your gut microbiome is an important in quieting the immune response, decreasing stress and anxiety, and reducing Hashimoto's flares.

While working on optimizing the gut microbiome, prescription medicines like SSRIs, which stands for serotonin reuptake inhibitors, or natural remedies, like 5-hydroxytryptophan or inositol (both used to enhance serotonin signaling), can help symptoms in the short term. L-glutamine, the precursor for glutamate, is sometimes also recommended to maintain healthy gut barrier function, while also helping regulate glutamate and GABA production. See the following table for dosage details.

TABLE 12.3. SUPPLEMENTS FOR ADRENAL AND GUT SUPPORT	
ADRENAL SUPPLEMENTS	RDA-SUGGESTED DOSING
B5	5 mg
B6	1.2–1.7 mg
B_{12}	2.4 mcg (but with B_{12} deficiency it is normally dosed at 500–1,000 mcg daily)
GUT SUPPLEMENTS	TYPICAL DOSING (NO RDA)
5-hydroxytryptophan	200–400 mg
Inositol	500–1,000 mg
L-glutamine	500–1,000 mg

Start low with dosing the gut supplements, if you choose to try one. Common side effects include headache, nausea, GI upset, and worsened anxiety or depression. Talk to your doctor and stop the supplements if you experience adverse reactions.

OUR ADVICE: Optimizing the gut microbiome through nutrition, vitamin support, and probiotics is of utmost importance in reducing stress, anxiety, and depression that contribute to Hashimoto's flares. If anxiety and depression is a component of your stress, consider discussing SSRI therapy with your doctor, or consider more natural approaches. If electing to try SSRI therapy or any of the natural supplements, monitor for worsening anxiety or depression and discontinue if these symptoms occur.

Optimizing the Liver
to Reduce Hashimoto's Flares

Like the adrenals and the gut, maintaining a healthy liver is also important. Think of the liver as your body's processing center. Within the liver, nutrients absorbed from your gut and from your foods are processed and stored for future use. In addition to processing nutrients, the liver also forms transport proteins—thyroid binding globulin (TBG), transthyretin, and albumin, which carry T4 and T3 to the tissues.

Finally, the liver is important in detoxifying environmental chemicals and drugs that could be harmful to the body. When the detoxification process isn't working well, environmental exposures that contribute to development of AITD accumulate within the body, worsening inflammation and the immune response. Just like most things in medicine, everyone is different and the effectiveness of these detoxification pathways can vary from person to person. Thankfully, there are some ways to optimize liver detoxification. Strategies include:

- limiting caffeine and alcohol

- limiting sugar and processed foods

- maintaining a healthy weight

- minimizing medications and supplements, particularly those that interact with each other

- reducing environmental exposures

- taking antioxidant vitamins (see Chapter 10 for details)

Although there are many liver detoxification cleanses and protocols to choose from, there are limited scientific studies to support their use. Instead, limiting exposures to harmful chemicals and medications while supporting detoxification pathways with nutritious foods and antioxidant vitamins is of utmost importance in maintaining optimal liver function. A healthy liver will be able to effectively eliminate harmful toxins, thereby reducing oxidative stress on the immune system, decreasing systemic inflammation, and improving immune function, all resulting in reduced Hashimoto's flares.

OPTIMIZING THYROID LEVELS

In addition to reducing Hashimoto's flares, one of the most important strategies in maintaining thyroid health is optimization of thyroid levels. During a Hashimoto's flare, thyroid levels can temporarily worsen and can contribute to worsening of AITD symptoms. Therefore, maintaining optimal thyroid levels is of utmost importance. There are a few tricks for optimizing levels that every thyroid patient should know. Here, you will find strategies that you can immediately integrate into your own treatment regimen to optimize your thyroid health.

Strategy 1. Take your thyroid medicine on an empty stomach.

We all know the instructions on the prescription bottle tell you to take the thyroid medicine thirty minutes to one hour from food and other medication. Although some patients can do this and consistently absorb the medication, a majority of people *cannot* fully absorb the medicine after only waiting thirty minutes.

In addition, caffeinated beverages, coffee creamer, calcium-fortified foods, high fiber foods, and other dairy products consumed too close to your thyroid medicine can dramatically decrease their absorption. When thyroid medicine is taken too close to these items, you will not consistently absorb the medicine. For example, instead of absorbing 100 percent of the medicine every day, you may be absorbing 50 percent on Monday, 80 percent on Tuesday, 70 percent on Wednesday, and so on—depending on what you've ingested. This inconsistent absorption of thyroid replacement medicine can leave you feeling like you are on a rollercoaster with your thyroid levels and may worsen AITD symptoms.

OUR ADVICE: Take your thyroid medicine every day on an empty stomach, spaced two hours from food and other medicine, and four hours from calcium or other vitamins. Make sure vitamins or prenatal vitamins are taken at least four hours from thyroid medication or at the opposite end of the day.

On the next page are the medications that most strongly interfere with thyroid absorption. Because many foods and medications interfere with absorption, it is best to take the thyroid medicine with water only at least two to four hours from these substances, or spaced at the opposite end of the day.

TABLE 12.4. MEDICATIONS THAT IMPACT THYROID ABSORPTION

MEDICATION TYPE	EXAMPLES
Antibiotics	Ciprofloxacin and other quinolone antibiotics such as Avelox and Levaquin.
Caffeine	Coffee, tea, colas, and energy drinks.
Calcium, iron, and magnesium	Coffee creamer, Ferrous sulfate, liquid iron, magnesium supplements, multivitamins, prenatal vitamins, slow Fe, and Tums.
Cholesterol-lowering medicines	Bile acid sequestrants, Colestid, Questran, Welchol, and Zetia.
Estrogen and SERMs	Birth control pills, Evista
Phosphorus binders	Renagel, Renvela
Stomach acid reducers	Antacids, Carafate, Prilosec, Protonix, Nexium, and Tums.

Strategy 2. Take your thyroid medicine at bedtime or in the middle of the night.

If you are on T4-only medicine, it is okay to move the medicine to bedtime, or take it when you get up in the middle of the night to use the restroom. This is particularly true if you find it difficult to wait a full two hours in the morning before eating or having your coffee. In fact, several studies have demonstrated better absorption at this time of day, because it is usually spaced two hours from food. It is more difficult to take T4/T3 combination therapy or T3 only therapy at bedtime because it can interfere with sleep. Therefore, if you're on any form of T3, it is best taken in the morning.

Strategy 3. Take your thyroid medicine every single day.

Missing just one or two doses in the month can dramatically affect your thyroid levels. Therefore, it is important to make sure that you take your medicine *every single day*. For patients that occasionally forget to take the medicine, there are a few strategies to ensure that you are taking your medicine as prescribed.

• Keep your medicine close by. This way, if you take it very early in the morning, you don't have to look around for it. This also helps cut down on forgetting to take it or remembering if you took it. Leave one pill out each night, and when it's gone the next day, you know you've taken it. No guess work involved.

- Set an alarm on your phone or other device to remind you to take the medicine.

- If you forget a dose, take it later that day—spaced appropriately from food and other medicine. It is okay to take the medicine at different times of the day as long as you're getting seven pills a week.

- Discuss with your doctor if he or she is okay with you doubling up on the thyroid medicine the next day if you forget to take a dose. Do not assume it is always safe to double up on missed doses, despite what you may have read or heard. While *typically* it is fine for most AITD patients to do this, you should still check with your doctor if you miss a dose.

Strategy 4. Maintain your weight.

Thyroid dosing is weight-dependent. This means that if you gain weight, you will most likely require an increased dose of your thyroid medicine. Conversely, if you lose weight, you will most likely need a decreased dose in your thyroid medicine. Typically, thyroid dosing changes if weight fluctuates 10 to 20 percent in either direction. Therefore, talk to your doctor if your weight significantly changes, as your medication dose may need to be adjusted.

Strategy 5. Check thyroid levels during various life stages.

Thyroid dosing can change during puberty, pregnancy, and menopause. It can also change after starting birth control pills or hormone replacement therapy. During these life-stages, make sure that you are working with your doctor to optimize your thyroid levels.

Strategy 6. Check the manufacturer.

Although less of an issue with name brand products, generic products can frequently change manufacturers. In this case, it is important to be aware of which pharmaceutical company manufactures your particular generic medicine and, if the manufacturer changes, monitor thyroid levels closely.

If you get compounded thyroid medicines, make sure that the starter com-pounded T4 or T3 isn't changed without your knowledge.

Strategy 7. Minimize interfering medications and supplements.

Keep your medicine and supplement list to a minimum. Work with your physician to determine if there are better choices in your medicine regimen that will not interfere with thyroid hormone metabolism. Refer to Chapter 5 for more details on interfering medicines.

Strategy 8. Work with your doctor when you feel "off."

Don't be afraid to ask to have your thyroid levels checked if you feel "off." Thyroid levels tend to worsen during Hashimoto's flares and sometimes for unidentified reasons. Check the expiration date on your thyroid medi-cine and consider refilling the prescription if you believe you have a "bad batch." You own thyroid gland can sometimes start producing thyroid hormone on its own, or can decrease its own thyroid hormone production to an even greater degree, necessitating changes in thyroid replacement dosing. Therefore, if you ever feel "off," *listen to your body* and ask to be tested.

CONCLUSION

Hashimoto's can be a frustrating disease, because there is a lot that is out of our control. However, as you now see, there are quite a few factors that we *can* influence in order to reduce flare-ups and optimize our thyroid func-tion. By avoiding your triggers when possible, improving your immune system, using thyroid replacement medication, decreasing inflammation, and increasing liver and gut function, you should find your AITD to be less active. While it is comforting to know that there are steps we can take to affect positive change with AITD, there are some people with Hashimoto's for whom more definitive steps must be taken. Next, we will explore the treatment options available to patients for whom monitoring and medica-tion is not enough.

13.

Treatments Beyond Medications

Sometimes, even after following the most perfect diet recommendations, adhering to proper supplements, and avoiding triggers, the immune system is just too damaged to be treated with a more conservative approach. Sometimes, people have had a strong viral trigger, a robust immune response, multiple autoimmune conditions, and have been dealing with symptoms for years. In these cases, more aggressive (also called definitive) therapy is needed.

When more aggressive therapy is necessary, it doesn't mean that the person has failed or hasn't persisted long enough in their quest for wellness—it just means that the disease is severe and that another therapy may work faster and more effectively. Many patients with severe AITD do not go into remission—and that's okay. In these situations, we have additional treatment options to optimize and regain thyroid health. Here we will discuss the three most common procedures used to treat Hashimoto's in detail, including medical indications, potential side effects, and expectations. These include:

- Radioactive iodine
- Ethanol ablation
- Surgery

WHEN TO CONSIDER OTHER TREATMENTS

If you're anything like us, as a doctor and patient, we both prefer to pursue the most natural and least aggressive treatment method first. Despite this, we also know that there is no one-size-fits-all approach to treating Hashimoto's, and that dietary changes and supplements can only go so far. Thankfully, most patients with typical AITD do not need more aggressive options. Others, however, including those with severe viral triggers, high viral loads and antibodies, longstanding AITD, continued exposure to triggers, or Hashitoxicosis, *do not* typically go into remission.

Additionally, patients with multiple autoimmune diseases who have been struggling for years to get well are also unlikely to enter remission. When considering definitive therapy, there are several questions to ask yourself:

1. Have you tried dietary and supplement recommendations for at least six to twelve months without effect?

2. Are you unable to follow strict dietary recommendations?

3. Are AITD symptoms disrupting your ability to function on a daily basis?

4. Have you been hospitalized for your thyroid symptoms?

5. Does your physician recommend definitive therapy based on your unique situation?

If you've answered "yes" to any of the above questions, this chapter is for you. If you are determined to pursue a more natural approach, it is still important to understand the advanced options that are available for you, should you need them in future.

RADIOACTIVE IODINE

After an entire chapter dedicated to avoiding environmental exposures and toxins, it may seem strange to present information on using a radioactive substance for treatment. But interestingly, small dose radioactive iodine therapy is a very effective *and safe* option for patients with severe Graves' disease, Hashitoxicosis with high uptake, toxic adenomas (or overactive thyroid nodules that cause hyperthyroidism), and certain types of advanced thyroid cancer. So what is radioactive iodine and how did we determine that it was useful in AITD?

Indications for Radioactive Iodine Use

Radioactive iodine, or RAI, is typically administered to patients as iodine-131 (I-131). This radiotracer is different than I-123 that is used for the thyroid uptake scan, as previously discussed. While I-123 is not radioactive and is only used for imaging, I-131 does have radioactive properties and is used as therapy to destroy abnormal thyroid tissue and thyroid cancer cells from the inside out.

The History of Radioactive Iodine

In 1936, two physicians by the name of Saul Hertz and Karl Compton were sitting together in a meeting when Dr. Hertz turned to Dr. Compton and asked whether iodine, which by this time had been identified as an important element for the thyroid, could be made radioactive to treat hyperthyroidism. Dr. Compton thought it could. Further research at the University of California, Berkeley identified two radioactive forms of iodine—iodine 130 and 131—as potential treatment candidates. In January 1941, Dr. Hertz was the first to administer radioactive iodine to a hyperthyroid patient at Massachusetts General Hospital—-and it was a success. But here's where the plot thickens.

Shortly after his discovery, Dr. Hertz joined the Navy Medical Corp during World War II and had to leave his work to a colleague, Dr. Earl Chapman. Upon returning home, Dr. Hertz realized that his research had been taken over completely by Dr. Chapman, leading to a fight over intellectual property and a major falling out between the two colleagues. Chapman, having had more time to perfect his research, wrote his paper first on the therapeutic effect of radioactive iodine in hyperthyroidism and sent it into the *Journal of the American Medical Association* (*JAMA*). While awaiting publication, Dr. Hertz got wind that Dr. Chapman was about to publish his paper and rushed to finish his own paper. Serendipitously, both papers were published in the same issue of *JAMA* on May 11, 1946, announcing radioactive iodine as a new, effective treatment for hyperthyroidism.

Since that time, tens of thousands of patients have undergone radioactive iodine therapy for hyperthyroidism and thyroid cancer. It has remained a very important treatment in patients who cannot attain spontaneous remission and has allowed many patients to avoid unnecessary surgical intervention.

There are currently several indications for the use of radioactive iodine treatment. These include:

- Graves' disease

- Hashitoxicosis with high thyroid uptake

- Thyroid cancer treatment after surgical intervention (in intermediate or high-risk patients only)

- Toxic adenoma, meaning a single thyroid nodule that is overactive or "hot," or toxic multinodular goiter, meaning many hot nodules, causing hyperthyroidism (also called Plummer's disease)

Is Radioactive Iodine Safe?

Radioactive iodine treatment has been around since the 1940s, much longer than many of the prescription drugs on the market. In typical treatment doses, particularly for AITD where the treatment doses are very low, it is extremely safe and effective. Most experts actually compare its safety to medications like aspirin. Although "radioactive" is in its name, it will *not* cause cancer, disease, or impair fertility when used at typical treatment doses for AITD or toxic nodules.

The half-life of radioactive iodine is about eight days, meaning that after eight days, the I-131 is half the strength of what was to start. It takes about five to ten half-lives (or forty to eighty days) for I-131 to completely deteriorate without a trace. Despite the time it takes to decay completely, radioactivity leaves the body completely within the first twenty-four to forty-eight hours, though sometimes radioactive precautions last seven to ten days after treatment, which we will discuss later in the chapter.

Despite its proven safety, there are several potential side effects that are important to be aware of. The most common side effect is hypothyroidism. When used for hyperthyroid patients, the goal of radioactive iodine is to destroy abnormally functioning thyroid tissue without surgery and render the patient hypothyroid. Once hypothyroid, lifelong thyroid replacement medicine will be needed to replace thyroid hormone for the nonfunctioning gland. In many cases, the I-131 treatment makes it much easier to definitively treat thyroid overactivity, normalize thyroid levels, and regain thyroid health. Other common side effects include anterior neck discomfort or swelling, and a metallic taste in the mouth that usually resolves after several days. Most patients have no side effects at all.

Less common side effects include a swelling of the glands on the sides of the face or under the jaw that help produce saliva, a condition called sialadenitis. This usually only occurs at high doses of I-131 used to treat thyroid cancer, not at the low doses used in AITD. The reason this happens is because I-131 concentrates not only in thyroid cells, but also in the salivary glands, disrupting the flow of saliva. Typical symptoms include facial swelling, redness of the skin, low-grade fever, a salty taste in mouth when eating, and facial or jaw pain. If you experience these symptoms, discuss them with your doctor.

Radioactive iodine can also rarely cause thyroiditis, or a destructive process within the thyroid gland that causes the thyroid to "spit out" extra thyroid hormones. This destructive thyroiditis can cause temporary worsening of hyperthyroidism in the weeks to months after treatment. If you notice worsening hyperthyroid symptoms after treatment, be sure to discuss them with your doctor.

Radioactive Iodine Treatment: What to Expect

If you and your doctor have determined that RAI is the best course of action for you, there are several things you should know before entering treatment. Specific recommendations will vary depending on your disease indication and individual recommendations from your doctor or nuclear medicine department. If you have questions or need clarification, do not be afraid to ask prior to treatment.

STEP 1: *Avoid Iodine or Anti-Thyroid Medicines Seven to Fourteen Days Prior to Treatment*

One of the most important things to do in preparation for RAI is to limit heavy iodine foods and stop anti-thyroid medicines like methimazole or propylthiouracil (PTU) seven to fourteen days prior to treatment. Although iodine is mostly found in fish, seaweed, and iodized salt, it can also be found in bread, dairy products, soy, egg yolks, canned foods, and restaurant foods. Following a low iodine diet (LID) is most important in patients with thyroid cancer, but should also be considered for AITD or hot thyroid nodules. The Thyroid Cancer Survivors' Association, Inc. (ThyCa) does an excellent job on recommendations for the low iodine diet and has an entire LID cookbook online. (See Resources on page 239.)

The thought behind avoiding iodine in the one to two weeks prior to treatment is that you are "starving" the abnormal thyroid cells from taking up iodine; because of this, the thyroid cells take up the radioactive iodine more readily and treatment may be more effective. The LID diet is not always required in AITD or toxic goiter, so be sure to discuss specific recommendations with your doctor.

STEP 2: *Complete a Thyroid Uptake Scan*

We already discussed the uptake scan in Chapter 6. (See page 78). As discussed, this scan does not typically use radioactive iodine, but instead I-123. The radiologists and nuclear medicine doctors use this scan to determine how much radioactive iodine is needed to treat the gland effectively.

If too little I-131 is administered, the treatment may fail and the patient may require repeat RAI or surgery. If too much I-131 is administered, side effects may be more common. Everyone is different, but a typical dose of radioactive iodine for AITD or toxic goiter ranges from 10 to 30 millicuries (mCi). Conversely, thyroid cancer patients can require upwards of 100 to 200 mCi and sometimes up to 1000 mCi, depending on the situation.

STEP 3: *Swallow the Radioactive Iodine*

Once it is determined that you are a candidate for RAI treatment, the nuclear medicine department will order the I-131 capsule or liquid from a certified pharmacy. Because I-131 decays with time, the treatment dose typically needs to be prepared the same day as treatment and delivered to the nuclear medicine department. Once delivered, you will be asked to swallow the radioactive iodine without touching it. Many times it is placed in a container to help assist with swallowing. You will then be given instructions on how many days to follow radioactive iodine precautions.

STEP 4: *Radioactive Iodine Precautions*

Although you are radioactive and must follow radioactive treatment precautions for a period of time, you are not so dangerous that you can't reenter society. If you have thyroid cancer and require very high doses of RAI, you may rarely need admission to the hospital overnight to allow your radioactivity counts to decrease to an acceptable level. Still, almost all patients will be discharged after treatment. Many of the recommendations after radioactive iodine are precautionary to prevent any significant exposure to your pets or your loved ones.

The two most significant populations at risk include pregnant women and children. We sometimes advise people to pretend like they have a severe cold and need to stay away from others. Radioactive iodine comes out in all bodily fluids, particularly in the first twenty-four to forty-eight hours. Therefore, we usually give the following precautions:

- *Stay out of public places and do not ride public transportation.* It is best to avoid restaurants, movies, shops, and other places where you will be around groups of people. The same is true of buses, trains, and planes. By avoiding close proximity to the public, you will not be exposing them to potential radiation.

- *Avoid pregnant women and children.* Maintain a distance of six feet from other adults. If you need to ride in the car with another adult, sit in the very back of the car, catty-corner to the driver.

- *Radioactive iodine is present in saliva and stomach fluids.* No kissing, sharing utensils, or sharing beverages. Buying paper plates, plastic silverware, and a disposable toothbrush that can be discarded at the end of the treatment period is advised. If you are easily nauseated, ask for anti-nausea medicine prior to swallowing the radioactive medicine to prevent vomiting.

- *Radioactive iodine is present in urine, stool, and menstrual products.* If you can do so, it is advisable to have your own bathroom during the precautionary period. If you cannot have your own bathroom, make sure that urine or stool is not present on the toilet seat. Men should sit down when urinating. Make sure that you flush the toilet bowl twice to remove any residual radioactive products. Individually dispose of any used tampons or pads.

- *Radioactive iodine is present in sweat and other bodily fluids.* Usually it is advised to sleep by yourself (that includes avoiding sleeping next to pets), because radioactive iodine can come out in sweat. It is also important to wash your own clothes and towels by themselves. Avoiding sex for at least one week after treatment is also advised.

For radioactive iodine used in AITD, radioactive iodine precautions usually only last one or two days. Some nuclear medicine department may even dismiss precautions because of the low dose that was given. In thyroid cancer, however, a much higher dose is usually administered, and precautions can last anywhere from five to ten days. Discuss your specific number of precautionary days with your doctor.

STEP FIVE: *Follow Up with Your Doctor*

As stated previously, most patients do not have any side effects in the days following treatment. Some patients can feel anterior neck pain or tightness.

Others can get post-therapy thyroiditis, resulting in transient worsening of hyperthyroidism. It is important to follow up with your doctor if you experience any of these symptoms. Additionally, in the six weeks to three months after therapy, it is important to frequently check thyroid levels so as to catch progression to hypothyroidism and start treatment. Work with your doctor closely in the weeks to months following therapy.

THYROID SURGERY

Surgery is another common form of definitive therapy for multiple thyroid diseases. In severe forms of AITD, patients can develop a very enlarged thyroid gland or goiter that causes compressive symptoms, including:

- choking sensation, particularly when laying on one's back

- difficulty swallowing

- pulling sensation at the base of the neck

- shortness of breath, chronic cough, or wheezing

- sleep apnea

These symptoms can occur because of other medical conditions as well, so discuss any symptoms with your doctor. If you are having thyroid compressive symptoms, you may wish to consider thyroid surgery. Additionally, if you have a thyroid nodule that is indeterminate with positive molecular testing, suspicious for thyroid cancer, or diagnostic of thyroid cancer, it is important to consider surgical intervention.

Unfortunately, it is not possible to remove the thyroid nodules themselves; instead, the full thyroid gland or thyroid lobe is removed. In special cases, it is possible to follow the suspicious nodules with serial ultrasound for growth instead of immediately pursuing surgery; if this course of action is pursued, make sure that you are seeing a very experienced thyroid doctor, preferably one that is ECNU-certified. (See Chapter 14.)

Prior to surgery, your doctor may wish to have a complete ultrasound done of the lymph nodes in your neck. This is important to determine the extent of surgical intervention and is called "lymph node mapping." Ask your doctor if this is needed prior to surgery.

Allison's Experience: Radioactive Iodine

I'm not going to sugar coat it—taking radioactive iodine was a weird experience. It wasn't painful or invasive. And it wasn't scary, at least to me. But it *was* strange. You have to swallow a capsule that you can't touch, because it's radioactive. I went home and followed all the precautions I was given. I didn't feel anything immediately after I swallowed it, or in the days that followed. A few weeks went by, and still nothing.

Then I started to feel sick. Really sick. As the radioactive iodine destroyed my thyroid, enormous amounts of hormones that had been stored in the gland were released into my body, a possible side effect called thyroiditis. I became extremely hyperthyroid, which occasionally happens with this treatment. Once Dr. Henderson helped me to get the excessive levels of thyroid hormone under control, I still felt a lot of pain and pressure in my throat and neck.

The radioactive iodine caused inflammation that made it feel tight and full around my throat and neck. It was unpleasant. I went for follow up ultrasounds to track my progress. I was nervous, didn't feel well, and doubted if I would ever feel better. Dr. Henderson encouraged me to remain hopeful and give it time. I did my best, but it was hard to be hopeful or patient when I felt so uncomfortable.

After a couple of months, I asked her to be brutally honest with me. Did she think there was any hope that I would feel better? Would the inflammation go down, as the nodules continued to shrink? She looked me in the eye and said she genuinely believed that I had a good chance of feeling better. She had seen this situation with other patients—some felt better quickly, while others had a rougher, extended experience.

A few weeks later, I did start to improve. Progress was slow and incremental, but progress is progress! Eventually, the tightness and pain relented, and as of today my thyroid nodules are *completely gone*. I can't say I haven't had any Hashimoto's flare-ups, but I can tell you that they aren't nearly as severe as before I had radioactive iodine treatment.

After thyroid treatment, I've had fewer flare-ups of my other autoimmune conditions, too. Before treatment, I was almost always in a flare-up of one or more conditions, including Hashimoto's. After everything settled down, I noticed that I wasn't getting the nearly constant flare-ups as before. Yes, I still get them (during times of other sickness, extreme stress, or lack of sleep), but they usually aren't as intense or lengthy. If anybody asked me if it was worth it, I wouldn't hesitate to tell them—*yes!*

Surgical Considerations

There are several considerations to be made prior to surgical treatment.

- **Find an experienced thyroid surgeon.** Studies have demonstrated that experience dramatically decreases your risk for surgical complications like hoarseness of voice or low calcium levels. Therefore, it is preferred that you undergo thyroid surgery with a surgeon that does *at least* twenty-five surgeries a year. Don't be afraid to ask about thyroid-specific surgical volumes.

- **Ask about the incision site.** One of the most common fears surrounding thyroid surgery is the scar on the neck. It is important that you discuss expectations with your surgeon prior to surgical intervention. This way, there'll be no surprises on the length and appearance of the incision. Although minimally invasive surgical techniques are available, there are multiple additional complications with these types of surgeries. After surgery, be sure to use sunscreen on the incision when you go outside. Alternatively, use a scarf to cover the incision when spending time in the sun. Additional topical therapies include commercially available scar treatment, vitamin E oil, and cocoa butter.

- **Ask about hospitalization and postoperative recovery.** Some centers are now moving towards outpatient surgery, meaning you can go home the same day. This is more typical in patients who only have one side of the thyroid removed. Ask your doctor about how long you might be in the hospital after surgery. Typically it is just one night. Although everyone is different with regard to postoperative recovery, most people are back at work within a week to ten days.

- **Make sure you are working with an experienced thyroid doctor after surgery.** Similar to radioactive iodine, thyroid replacement therapy is needed many times after thyroid surgery. If you only had a portion of the thyroid removed, you may not need replacement medicine. Otherwise, make sure you have a game plan with regard to optimal thyroid dosing after surgery. Find a thyroid doctor that is an expert at thyroid dosing and titration. Most of the time, you will be started on thyroid replacement medicine during hospitalization and go home on the medicine. You should follow up with your thyroid doctor four to eight weeks after surgery to check your thyroid dosing and ensure that it is correct.

ALTERNATIVES TO SURGERY

If you have a thyroid cyst or thyroid cancer, there are some cutting-edge treatments available that allow select patients to avoid surgery. In appropriate cases, fluid-filled thyroid cysts and recurrent thyroid cancer lymph nodes can be treated with less invasive alternatives. Because these techniques are relatively new, they are not yet universally available, so be sure to check online to see if these options are available in your area.

■ ETHANOL ABLATION THERAPY

Ethanol ablation therapy (also called percutaneous ethanol injection, or PEI) is a treatment that can be used to shrink large thyroid cysts and fluid-filled nodules, as well as destroy recurrent thyroid cancer lymph nodes without surgical intervention. Ethanol ablation is a relatively painless technique similar to fine needle aspiration biopsy, where ethanol is injected into the cyst or cancerous lymph node, thereby destroying the blood supply to the lesion. There are minimal side effects and risks, making ethanol ablation therapy a very effective definitive treatment in certain circumstances. A majority of patients treated for thyroid cysts do not require a replacement thyroid medicine after treatment. Preparation steps before, during, and after the procedure are similar to that of thyroid FNA biopsy; refer to Chapter 7 for details on how to prepare.

Key Points About Ethanol Ablation Therapy

- There may be minimal discomfort associated with the procedure.

- Typically, ethanol ablation is a onetime-only procedure, though sometimes multiple treatment sessions are needed.

- Usually, there are little to no side effects, with the exception of slight soreness at the procedure site. Rare side effects include neck swelling, short-term voice hoarseness, worsened AITD, and low-grade fever.

- Patients are typically asked to refrain from heavy lifting (over 25 lbs), particularly overhead, for twenty-four to forty-eight hours after the procedure.

■ Radiofrequency Ablation (RFA)

Radiofrequency ablation (RFA) is another minimally invasive technique that uses a probe the size of a needle to shrink thyroid nodules using alternating frequencies and heat. The technique has been long used in Europe and Asia, but is relatively new in the United States. Nodules can decrease in size by 30 to 80 percent, depending on the type of nodule. Most patients do not require thyroid medicine after the procedure, and there are few side effects. Preparation steps before, during, and after the procedure are similar to that of thyroid FNA biopsy; refer to Chapter 7 for details on how to prepare. Patients may be asked to remain NPO (nothing to eat after midnight) for the procedure, and may be given light anesthesia sedation, similar to what is given for a colonoscopy procedure.

■ High-Intensity Focused Ultrasound (HIFU) Ablation

Another non-operative technique for benign solid thyroid nodules is high intensity focused ultrasound (HIFU). This form of minimally invasive treatment uses focused ultrasound waves to destroy benign thyroid nodules through the skin, without the use of needles. Nodules have been shown to shrink by an average of 50 percent in volume, but do not go away completely. Treatment is currently only available in Europe.

Commonalities of Non-Surgical Techniques

When appropriate, both ethanol ablation and high intensity focused ultrasound ablation are techniques that allow patients to forego surgery and avoid the need for thyroid replacement medicine. Non-operative techniques are still an emerging treatment area. While they are a viable option for some, and are gaining in use, they are not yet widely available. Talk with your doctor to determine if you would qualify for non-invasive technologies.

WHAT TO EXPECT FROM TREATMENTS BEYOND MEDICATION

As with every other aspect of patients' thyroid experiences, no two people are exactly the same. Most patients will have excellent results after undergoing the treatments we have covered, while others will not have complete and total success. Most patients who pursue these treatments do find a significant level of improvement. Some patients who undergo more treatment options, like radioactive iodine or surgery, have a more difficult time regaining thyroid health after the procedure. Therefore, it is essential to establish good communication with your thyroid healthcare provider.

It is important to work closely with your provider when discussing both non-surgical and surgical options. Working with an experienced thyroid doctor who is willing to try different thyroid replacement options and actively titrate your thyroid medicine to optimize thyroid health after treatment is of utmost importance. With open, clear communication and a team-based approach, you and your healthcare provider can discuss concerns, expectations, and questions every step of the way.

CONCLUSION

As you can see, there are different approaches when it comes to treatments beyond medication for AITD, nodules, and cancer. It is of the utmost importance that you choose a doctor who is familiar with all therapeutic options, including the most current.

You've read a lot of information thus far. Probably there have been times along the way where it has seemed overwhelming. That is totally understandable. The AITD journey is not a quick or easy one. But you are already further along than when you started this book. Now you have more knowledge than you did before. But where do you go from here? In the final chapter, we will help you to figure out how to approach your search for a provider and how and where to find pertinent, credible information moving forward.

14.

Moving Forward

Now that you've read about the many aspects of Hashimoto's, including the symptoms, testing, diagnosis, related conditions, the variety of treatments, and how to manage Hashimoto's flare-ups, you're probably wondering where you go from here. Maybe you want to start your search for a qualified medical provider to give you a second opinion or guide you on your journey with autoimmune thyroid disease. Or perhaps you want to explore additional sources of information. Possibly you feel overwhelmed by Hashimoto's and wonder if people can actually improve. In this chapter, we'll take you through the best ways to find doctors and information, as well as provide some inspiring and hopeful success stories!

WHY IS IT SO HARD TO FIND THE RIGHT DOCTOR?

Thyroid disease in general, and Hashimoto's specifically, is something that many providers shy away from. Why? Most doctors want to help their patients, but they are results-driven, meaning they want to find a treatment or cure for their patients as quickly and effectively as possible. As you now know, AITD doesn't work that way. Everything about it is time-consuming from both the patient and physician perspective. It takes time and persistence to arrange and undergo the necessary testing and diagnostic procedures—as well as the commitment needed to figure out the best treatment. This usually means tweaking and modifying treatment along the way in order to help patients achieve and maintain their best possible thyroid health.

Because Hashimoto's patients require a significant amount of time and attention, most primary care physicians simply don't have the time to spend with what is considered "high-maintenance" patients, nor do they

typically have the time or interest to develop an in-depth understanding of thyroid issues. Endocrinologists are more familiar with thyroid issues, since they specialize in a variety of endocrine gland and hormone disorders.

However, even these specialists don't always have comprehensive, wide ranging knowledge of Hashimoto's. Many endocrinologists have a practice that is primarily focused on diabetes, while others concentrate on adrenal, pituitary, or reproductive issues. If you have AITD, it's advisable to work with a thyroid specialist—and yes, there is such a thing. These doctors have extensive education and training in thyroid disease and thyroid cancer. It can be challenging to find such a physician, but it is possible.

FINDING A THYROID SPECIALIST

A basic Google search will return a seemingly endless supply of health practitioners who advertise themselves as thyroid specialists. These thyroid specialists come from many training backgrounds and include chiropractors (DC), naturopaths (ND), general practitioners (MD/DO/NP/PA), integrative medicine practitioners (any of the above initials), and endocrinologists (MD/DO). No matter what type of thyroid specialist you choose to work with, it is extremely important that you inquire as to their education, training, and experience treating patients with AITD.

There are wide ranges of healthcare providers who treat thyroid patients. Remember, almost anyone in the health services field can claim to specialize in AITD/Hashimoto's. Maybe they have undergone extensive training about thyroid issues through continuing education. Or maybe they only took a one-time seminar for a couple of hours. Formal medical training can be as short as two years or as long as ten years for specialty-trained endocrinologists. (See Table 14.1 on page 204 for more details.) The responsibility is yours to be an informed patient. When searching online for the right thyroid doctor, you can Google potential doctors' names to learn more about their medical training and experience with Hashimoto's. Once you've found a provider who seems like the right fit, take time at your appointments to ask questions regarding his or her thyroid knowledge, training, and experience.

On the following page, Table 14.1 lists the most common types of thyroid providers along with specifics on their credentials and training.

TABLE 14.1. MEDICAL CAREGIVERS' CREDENTIALS		
INITIALS	**TITLE**	**TRAINING**
D.C.	Doctor of Chiropractic	4 years chiropractic school
D.O.	Doctor of Osteopathy	4 years medical school plus 3 to 5 years residency +/– 2 to 3 years fellowship
M.D.	Medical Doctor	4 years medical school plus 3 to 5 years residency +/– 2 to 3 years fellowship
N.D.	Doctor of Naturopathy	4 years of naturopathic school
N.P.	Nurse Practitioner	Registered nurse plus 2 years graduate degree in nursing practice
P.A.	Physician Assistant	2 to 3 years physician assistant program

Let's look a little closer at the types of providers to consider when seeking a partner in your Hashimoto's care. Just like with all the previous aspects of AITD we have discussed, there is no one-size-fits-all approach. Some patients feel most comfortable with a conventional MD, while others may find an integrative approach is better for them. What is *most* important is to find someone who is sufficiently qualified to treat patients with AITD.

Endocrinologists

An endocrinologist is a medical doctor who specializes in the glands and hormones related to the endocrine system. They have either gone through traditional medical school or an osteopathic medical school, have completed a residency in internal medicine, and have finished (typically) a two or three year fellowship of specialized training in endocrinology. They diagnose and treat thyroid disorders, diabetes, metabolic disorders, osteoporosis, and adrenal gland conditions. Some endocrinologists continue their education and training in order to specialize in one area of endocrinology, such as AITD.

If you want to find an endocrinologist (a medical doctor) who specializes in thyroid disease, there are several ways to conduct a search. The American Thyroid Association (ATA) and The American Association of Clinical Endocrinologists (AACE) are credible resources, both with websites (in the Resources section) where you can search for a thyroid specialist.

Another option is a website where patients write reviews of doctors. This free, user-friendly website allows you to search for endocrinologists within a geographical area of your choosing. The site provides important information, including doctor ratings on a scale from one to five stars, and patient experiences. Links to the doctors' websites are typically included, so you can read more about them and access contact info.

Many doctors are not willing to do other blood tests beyond TSH. Unbelievably, this is true even of some endocrinologists. You might find resistance if you suggest a more comprehensive panel of tests. An endocrinologist who is a thyroid specialist, however, will be very familiar with the range of tests available. Most likely, not only will they will be willing to order them, they'll *want* to order them, because they understand the valuable information that will result. An endocrinologist who is a thyroid specialist will typically have at least 40 percent of their practice devoted to thyroid disease and thyroid cancer. Do not be afraid to ask.

Since endocrinologists practice within the traditional medical system, they are more likely to take insurance when compared to some other practitioners. This is usually the case when they are part of a teaching hospital or university medical center. However, there are some endocrinologists who may operate a private practice and chose not to accept insurance. It is always best to inquire.

ECNU-Certified Endocrinologists

As we previously discussed, ultrasound is a critical diagnostic tool when it comes to thyroid nodules, associated with AITD and thyroid cancer. Regardless of what medical procedure you must undergo, it's wise to choose a practitioner who has a lot of experience performing this procedure. You don't want to go to someone who does an ultrasound occasionally. There are thyroid specialists who have undergone specialized training through The American Association of Clinical Endocrinologists to gain certification, known as ECNU—which stands for endocrine certification in neck ultrasound.

When you go to an ECNU-certified endocrinologist, you are able to have your ultrasound right at their office/facility. No running around to various locations. Another advantage is that when they do repeat ultrasounds over time, they have the previous ones to reference for changes. This is similar to what's done if you go to the same place for a yearly mammogram. In that case, a radiologist compares what has remained consistent, and what might have changed. Your ECNU endocrinologist does this same thing, only they discuss it with you right there. No waiting for a phone call or letter. Typically, they will tell you directly what they saw.

Integrative/Functional Medicine Providers, Naturopaths, and Chiropractors

There are some integrative/functional medicine providers, naturopaths, and chiropractors who are also knowledgeable about AITD. Skilled functional and integrative medicine providers incorporate nutrition and diet to help patients optimize their health, which is something conventional medical practitioners are not typically as interested in or informed about. Chiropractors may be more skilled at treating muscle pain and joint pain associated with AITD. All of these providers base their patient care on a comprehensive approach, where they try to figure out the underlying cause of the medical problem—rather than just giving patients something to treat it. This type of provider is usually interested in incorporating nutritional supplements and diet into treatment plans. While these healthcare providers may be more willing to do more extensive testing than conventional doctors, they commonly don't take insurance. This could lead you to inadvertently incur considerable financial expenses for visits and tests. Vitamins and supplements may also come with additional cost.

Although there are providers with formal thyroid-specific medical training in the fields of functional/integrative medicine and chiropractic medicine, there are others who do not have the same level of rigorous medical training. Be an informed healthcare consumer and ask!

So Who is Right for Me?

It can be a little confusing deciding what type of provider to seek. Both physicians and others, including chiropractors, naturopaths, homeopaths, nutritionists, and acupuncturists, can refer to themselves as "integrative" or "functional" medicine providers. Physicians can be either MDs or DOs, and they may or may not consider themselves to be practicing functional or integrative medicine. You may actually need to see more than one provider to optimize thyroid health. Sometimes patients need an endocrinologist for medication control, but also choose to see an alternative health provider for diet/nutrition needs.

There are certain things to look for, and others to avoid, when seeking a provider. Look for a provider who:

- checks to see if you have nutritional deficiencies.

- expresses a willingness to discuss your case with the other providers you may be seeing.

- has a practice with at least 40 percent devoted to thyroid patients, preferably more.

- is willing to be flexible about modifying your treatment, if you need to.

- listens to what you have to say.

- offers reasonable expectations about what they can do for you.

- uses a range thyroid specific blood test to make sure your levels are optimized.

Avoid a provider who:

- does not have specific training in thyroid issues.

- ignores your feedback about how you are reacting to treatment.

- insists that that you need many types of supplements, without proof of deficiency.

- insists you follow a gluten free, vegetarian, paleo, or any other specific type of diet without discussing your specific circumstances.

- refuses to order crucial thyroid tests.

- tries to sell you expensive supplements.

Provider Care Services

Different providers can offer different services. It is important to understand what a provider can and cannot do for you in the course of your care. Table 14.2 details the specifics of various providers and the services they are able to offer. Keep in mind that just because they can provide a service, does not mean that they do. Look at their website, read patient reviews, and call their offices and ask questions.

	CHIRO-PRACTOR (DC)	ENDO-CRINOLOGIST (MD OR DO)	INTEGRATIVE/ FUNCTIONAL PROVIDER (MD OR DO)	NATUROPATH (ND)	NURSE PRACTITIONER (NP)	PHYSICIAN ASSISTANT (PA)
TABLE 14.2. SERVICES BY PROVIDER						
Diet counseling	X	X	X	X	X	X
Ethanol ablation and other advanced techniques		Sometimes				
Nutrition counseling	X	X	X	X	X	X
Nutritional deficiency testing	X	X	X	X	X	X
Prescribe medication		X	X	Varies by state	X	X
Order RAI treatment		X				
Supplement sales	X	X	X	X	X	X
Thyroid biopsy		Sometimes				
Thyroid blood testing	X	X	X	X	X	X
Thyroid ultrasound		Sometimes	Few		Few	Few

NOT ALL INFORMATION IS CREATED EQUAL

As we've stated from the beginning, the amount of information out there can be overwhelming, and even paralyzing. As you continue to seek knowledge about Hashimoto's, it's important to remember that just because someone claims something on a website, blog, or message board doesn't mean that it's true. That doesn't necessarily mean that it's dishonest, either. When people who suffer from Hashimoto's, or any other medical problem, for that matter, find something that they believe helps them, they're understandably enthusiastic about it. Whether it's a health provider, a special diet, certain supplements, medications, or alternative or traditional treatments, people want to share it with others. And while it can be helpful to read about other Hashimoto's patients' experiences, you should have a discerning eye.

Although Hashimoto's patients share similar struggles and can find valuable support among the Hashimoto's community, everyone is an individual with their own specific medical needs. Just as there is no one-size-fits-all approach to thyroid supplementation, there isn't one universal Hashimoto's experience. What works for someone else, may not work for you. However, if you uncover the same information from multiple sources, and it's something you think you may want to pursue, you should discuss it with your doctor.

Finally, you may want to explore other books about Hashimoto's, autoimmune disease, or thyroid dysfunction, gut health, or alternative treatments. Perhaps you already have. As you read, it's prudent to always consider the source of the information. Again, this doesn't mean that the information provided is "wrong" or "untrue." It simply means that if an author's background is one of hormones, or chiropractic medicine, or low carb diets, or the author supports one type of thyroid replacement and is completely against all others—you must consider the source. If someone has a vested interest in following one plan, one method, one lifestyle, or one treatment, that is going to be reflected in their writing. It's absolutely fine to expose yourself to varying points of view and different perspectives. Just do so with the awareness that what you're reading may be trying to convince you that their way is the *only* way.

Be skeptical of anything that sounds like a miracle treatment or cure. Likewise, it's best to avoid websites, blogs, and books that use scare tactics, warning you of horrible things that will happen to you if you fail to follow their recommendations.

HAVING REALISTIC EXPECTATIONS

It's a challenge to have any kind of autoimmune disease, and that includes Hashimoto's. But with proper diagnosis and treatment, patients can and do improve. For some, the improvement happens quickly. They get on a thyroid replacement that works well for them and their levels stay relatively stable, without requiring much tweaking. If they're deficient in certain vitamins or minerals, they take the necessary supplements. Maybe they find out they have to make dietary changes, in addition to other aspects of maintaining good thyroid health. For other patients, the journey to feeling better isn't so straightforward, but working with their doctor, they eventually find their health improving.

The process of finding the right provider, having all necessary testing, getting diagnosed, and trying various treatment approaches can be a

Allison's Experience: Two Steps Forward, One Step Back

Success isn't always linear. Sometimes you're making strides, only to have a setback. Sometimes the setbacks are small; sometimes quick. Other times, they're major and last a while. You might start wondering, even worrying, if it'll be permanent. At least that's been my experience. As I mentioned earlier, my various autoimmune related illnesses tend to work collectively. They flare up together, one triggering the next, and the next . . . you get the idea. When there's a period of abatement, not only does my Hashimoto's become very dormant, but typically so does my CFS and Fibro.

Conversely, when any one of those conditions kick starts my immune system into high gear, a chain reaction gets triggered. It could be lack of sleep, getting sick, stress, weather conditions, and an endless list of other variables. Some of these are completely out of my control, while others I can directly influence. If I slack off on the supplements I'm lacking in, it doesn't take long to feel a flare creeping up. I don't like to think of myself as having AITD, or any other illness, so sometimes I push myself too hard. And I always pay for it afterward.

Let's be real: It's not fun having to deal with medical issues. But you know what's worse? Not dealing with them. Giving up on finding the right medical care. Not putting in the effort to get to reach your own personal best. I've learned that with great medical care, and consistently doing my part by taking

time-consuming process. It will serve you better to have realistic expectations of reaching improved thyroid health, rather than expecting a miracle, quick fix, or magic bullet. There is no reason to believe that you can't find improvement with proper care and effective management of your Hashimoto's.

CONCLUSION

Seeking out information, filtering out what's not credible, and trying to understand what has value can all be tiring and frustrating. This is especially true when you're not feeling well and don't have much energy. Again, this is where a thyroid specialist comes in. As a partner in your thyroid health, their work doesn't end when you get a diagnosis. It doesn't medications, supplements, and getting enough sleep, it is possible to have better days.

Everyone must define success for themselves. For me, there is a certain way I'm used to feeling. It's not what I would call "healthy." There are every-day aspects of my various medical conditions that make themselves known through a variety of symptoms. Over the years, I've gotten used to this. It's what I consider my baseline. Maybe you have one too. You might not feel great, but you feel a way that you are used to and can deal with. Then a day comes when things get ramped up, into a flare-up of some type. I try to stay calm and remind myself that this too shall pass. And it does.

Sometimes, occasionally, I even have short periods where I feel slightly better than my baseline! Even though those times are brief, they are incredibly uplifting. I know they are temporary, but the fact that there are moments or hours such as this gives me hope. *That* feels like success. When a flare-up subsides, *that* feels like success. When I go one day longer than usual without a really bad day, *that* feels like success. And when I'm not doing well and talk to my doctor—and she not only listens, but works to help figure out what's going on and how to address it—*that* feels like success.

Any control you can take over your health means *you* are having success. Be kind to yourself and try to resist the urge to get overwhelmed, frustrated, and down about setbacks. You're on the right path. You will most likely have times when your progress sputters, slows down, or even temporarily stops. That's okay. You just have to keep going.

end when they prescribe that first thyroid replacement medication, or when you adjust your supplements or diet. It also doesn't end the minute you start to feel improvement. The relationship remains fluid, changing and adapting to your needs along the way.

There will be times when you feel "off," indicating your AITD is flaring up. Or maybe your thyroid hormone levels are slightly low, or high. You might need to change medications or add something to your regimen. Maybe you'll read something on the Internet and need your doctor's perspective on it. Choose wisely when selecting a provider. If you don't feel as if they are in it with you, find someone else. That's easier said than done, but it's worth the effort to find the right person. Make sure it's someone you feel comfortable with as you continue your journey.

Conclusion

As a doctor specializing in thyroid problems and a patient suffering from Hashimoto's disease, we both understand where you are right now—whether you're just starting out and trying to determine if your symptoms are from Hashimoto's, or you've been through a comprehensive diagnostic process and are undergoing treatment. Others have felt the physical and mental exhaustion of dealing with AITD, too. They've been frustrated by dealing with medical providers who either don't believe them, refuse to order the requested blood work, or won't take their medication preferences into consideration.

There *are* people with Hashimoto's who have gotten the care they need. They've had sustained periods of feeling better. They've gone from being immobilized and unable to function normally, to again being productive and active. They've regained hope. It's possible!

Remember, Hashimoto's is not something you are born with, and it's not an illness that you can catch. It is a response by your body to factors such as illness, environmental factors, and genetics, which causes an autoimmune response. You can't always "cure" it, or get rid of it completely. Even if you do enter remission, you may experience a relapse months or years down the road. But with the correct treatment, you can have many better days, and fewer bad days, where your Hashimoto's is active and making you feel sick, in pain, or exhausted.

All the information in this book is designed to help you to be aware of the many aspects of AITD, in an effort to help you achieve better thyroid health. Because better thyroid health means better overall health. But there is one thing that is the most important factor in your thyroid journey—and that is *you!*

You are the best expert when it comes to your health. *You* are the one who will know first if you feel "off," or are beginning a flare-up. *You* know if a medication doesn't feel right for you. Because each of us may react differently when doing the exact same things to address our symptoms, you will find that no singular treatment works for everyone. Therefore, the only way you can improve is if you consistently advocate for your thyroid health. Nobody else can do this for you, which is why you must remain observant, attentive, and involved with the treatment(s) of your AITD. This is true every step of the way, up to and including after you get your Hashimoto's well controlled.

You've already taken a great first step towards achieving that goal by reading this book. But this is just the beginning. You must remain proactive in your quest to feel (and remain) better. As you travel on your Hashimoto's journey, we wish you a life full of love, laughter, and good thyroid health. Our sincere desire is that each of you can move from being a Hashimoto's sufferer—to someone *living with* and *living well* with Hashimoto's.

Glossary

Antibody. A large protein produced by cells in the blood in response to antigens that the body normally does not recognize, such as bacteria, viruses, and any substance the body senses as foreign. As part of the body's immune system, antibodies are designed to attack these types of antigens.

Antigen. Any triggering substance that is identified by the body that induces a response by the immune system.

ATA. American Thyroid Association.

Autoimmunity. The misdirection of the body's immune response, resulting in an attack on one's own healthy cells.

Autoimmune thyroid disease (AITD). An autoimmune disorder in which antibodies attack the thyroid gland. AITD can be diagnosed as either Hashimoto's or Graves' Disease.

Biopsy. A sample of cells that are removed from the body and used for diagnostic purposes.

Definitive therapy. A treatment that is intended to bring about a specific cure. These are more aggressive than a medication-only approach.

Deiodinases. Enzymes that convert to the thyroid hormones T4 to T3.

Endocrine system. The group of glands which secrete hormones that help to coordinate and control all metabolic activities in our body. These glands include the adrenal glands, parathyroid gland, pituitary gland, and thyroid gland, in addition to the ovaries, pancreas, and testes.

Endocrinologist. A doctor who specializes in disorders/diseases of the endocrine system and associated hormones.

GMO. Genetically modified organism. This term normally refers to foods whose genetic composition have been altered, however it can also refer various microorganisms.

Graves' disease. An inflammatory autoimmune disease of the thyroid, resulting in hyperthyroidism.

Halogenated. Chemicals that contains halogen atoms. These include bromine, chlorine, fluorine, or iodine. "Halogen" means "salt producing," because when combined with metal, they produce a variety of salts.

Hashimoto's thyroiditis. Also known as Hashimoto's Disease. An inflammatory autoimmune disease of the thyroid, resulting in hypothyroidism.

Hashitoxicosis. Hyperthyroidism caused by Hashimoto's.

Hyperthyroidism. A condition in which the thyroid produces too much thyroid hormone.

Hypothyroidism. A condition in which the thyroid produced too little thyroid hormone.

H. Pylori. A type of bacteria found in the stomach, typically responsible for the majority of stomach ulcers.

Iodide. The ion state of iodine, which occurs when iodine bonds with another element. When we ingest foods with iodine, a biochemical process then converts that iodine into its absorbable form: iodide. This is how we get a usable form of the necessary iodine needed for thyroid function.

Iodine. An element needed to produce necessary amounts of T4 and T3. Since the body does not produce iodine, it must be ingested through food consumption.

Microbiome. An ecosystem consisting of the collective set of microbes that live in or on the human body. The greatest concentration of bacteria is in our digestive system, called "gut microbiome."

Nodule. A fluid-filled or solid lump or bump found in or on our bodies. Nodules can indicate a fluid collection, and immune reaction, or an overgrowth of cells.

Nutrient. Substances that provide any living organism with nourishment to carry on all life-sustaining processes. These include carbohydrates, fats, minerals, proteins, vitamins, and water.

Nutritional Supplement. Also called dietary supplements, these are usually taken orally, and are used to enhance nutrients we are lacking. These include amino acids, minerals, proteins, and vitamins.

Phytoestrogens. Naturally occurring compounds found in certain plants, which can affect the body's estrogen levels.

Pituitary gland. A pea-sized gland that is located at the base of the brain. Also called the "Master Gland" because it controls several hormones, including TSH.

Subclinical hyperthyroidism. A condition in which the thyroid overproduces thyroid hormone, but is not indicated on T3 or T4 lab tests, although it does affect TSH levels.

Subclinical hypothyroidism. A condition in which the thyroid underproduces thyroid hormone, but is not indicated on T3 or T4 lab tests, although it does affect TSH levels.

T3. Triiodothyronine.

T4. Thyroxine.

Tg. Thyroglobulin.

TBG. Thyroxine-binding globulin.

Thyroglobulin (Tg). A protein produced by the thyroid. The presence of Tg antibodies typically suggests Hashimoto's thyroiditis, and less frequently, Graves' disease. Tg is measured in thyroid cancer patients as a way to follow disease progression.

Thyroxine (T4). The inactive form of thyroid hormone, accounting for 80 percent of all thyroid hormones.

Thyroxine-binding globulin (TBG). A protein which helps move thyroid hormones into the bloodstream.

Thyroid Peroxidase (TPO). An enzyme associated with thyroid hormone production. The presence of TPO antibodies suggests autoimmune thyroid disease (AITD).

Thyroid stimulating hormone (TSH). A hormone that is produced by the pituitary gland. TSH prompts the thyroid to produce thyroxine (T4), which is then converted to triiodothyronine (T3).

TPO. Thyroid Peroxidase.

Triiodothyronine (T3). The active form of thyroid hormone, which works to regulate metabolism, heart rate and body temperature.

TSH. Thyroid-stimulating hormone.

Ultrasound. A diagnostic imaging test that uses high frequency sound waves.

References

Chapter 1

Bahn RS, Burch HB, Cooper DS Garber JR, Greenlee MC, Klein I, Laurberg P, McDougall IR, Montori VM, Rivkees SA, Ross, DS, Sosa JA, Stan MN. Hyperthyroidism and Other Causes of Thyrotoxicosis: Management Guidelines of the American Thyroid Association and American Association of Clinical Endocrinologists. 2011 Endocr Pract;17(3).

Garber JR, Cobin RH, Gharib H, Hennessey JV, Klein I, Mechanick JI, Pessah-Pollack R, Singer PA, Woeber KA. Clinical Practice Guidelines for Hypothyroidism In Adults: Cosponsored by the American Association of Clinical Endocrinologists and the American Thyroid Association. 2012 Endocr Pract;18(6).

Hollowell JG, Staehling NW, Flanders WD, et al. Serum TSH, T4, and thyroid antibodies in the United States population (1988 to 1994): National Health and Nutrition Examination Survey (NHANES III). 2002 J Clin Endocrinol Metab 87(2):489-499.

Kim DW, Jung SL, Baek JH, et al. The prevalence and features of thyroid pyramidal lobe, accessory thyroid and ectopic thyroid as assessed by computed tomography: a multicenter study. 2013 Thyroid;23(1):84-91.

Spencer CA, Hollowell JG, Kazarosyan M, Braverman LE. National Health and Nutrition Examination Survey III thyroid stimulating homorne (TSH)-thyroperoxidase antibody relationships demonstrate that TSH upper reference limits may be skewed by occult thyroid dysfunction. 2007 J Clin Endocrinol Metab; 92(11):4236-40.

Chapter 2

American Cancer Society. Cancer Facts & Figures 2018 [Internet]. American Cancer Society; 2018. Available from: https://www.cancer.org/content/dam/cancer-org/research/cancer-facts-and-statistics/annual-cancer-facts-and-figures/2018/cancer-facts-and-figures-2018.pdf

Amino, N., Tada, H., Hidaka, Y., & Hashimoto, K. Hashimoto's disease and Dr. Hakaru Hashimoto. 2002 Endocrine Journal. 2002; 49(4), 393.

Armelagos GJ, Harper K. The Paleolithic Disease-scape, the Hygiene Hypothesis, and the Second Epidemiological Transition. In: Rook GAW, The Hygiene Hypothesis and Darwinian Medicine. 2009 Birkhauser Basel;29-43.

Bignell GR, Canzian F, Shayeghi M, Stark M, Shugart YY, Biggs P, Mangion J, Hamoudi R, Rosenblatt J, Buu P, Sun S, Stoffer SS, Goldgar DE, Romeo G, Houlston RS, Narod SA, Stratton

MR, Foulkes WD. Familial nontoxic multinodular thyroid goiter locus maps to chromosome 14q but does not account for familial nonmedullary thyroid cancer. 1997 Am J Hum Genet;61:1123-1130.

Braun-Fahlander, C et al. Prevalence of Hay Fever and Allergic Sensitization in Farmers' Children and Their Peers Living in the Same Rural Community. 1999 Clin Exp Allergy:29(1).

Braun-Fahrlander C et al. Environmental Exposure to Endotoxin and Its Relation to Asthma in School-Age Children. 2002 N Engl J Med: 247(2).

Columbia University Dept of Surgery. http://columbiasurgery.org/news/2015/09/03/history-medicine-leonardo-da-vinci-and-elusive-thyroid-0

Dean DS, Gharib H. Epidemiology of thyroid nodules. 2008 Best Pract Res Clin Endocrinol Metab;22(6):901-11.

Douwes J, et al. Farm Exposure In Utero May Protect Against Asthma, Hay Fever and Eczema. 2008 Eur Respir.J:(32)3:603-11.

Emanuel MB. Hay Fever, a Post Industrial Revolution Epidemic: A History of Its Growth During the 19th Century. 1988 Clin Exp Allergy:18(3).

Hoffman K, Lorenzo A, Butt CM, Hammel SC, Henderson BB, Roman SA, Scheri RP, Stapleton HM, Sosa JA. Exposure to flame retardant chemicals and occurrence and severity of papillary

thyroid cancer: A case-control study. 2017 Environ Int;107:235-242.

Kimball OP, Marine D Nutrition. The prevention of simple goiter in man. Second paper. 1918. 1992 Nutrition;8(3):200-4.

Knobel M, Medeiros-Neto G. An outline of inherited disorders of the thyroid hormone generating system. 2003 Thyroid;13:771-80.

Lydiatt DD, Bucher GS. Historical vignettes of the thyroid gland. Clin Anat. 2011 Jan;24(1):1-9

Markel H. "When it rains it pours:" endemic goiter, iodized salt, and David Murray Cowie, MD. 1987 Am J Public Health;77(2):219-29.

Merke F. History of endemic cretinism. In: History and Iconography of Endemic Goiter and Cretinism. Berne: Hans Huber Publishers; 1984.

Mitman G. Hay Fever Holiday: Health, Leisure, and Place in Gilded Age America. 2003 Bull Hist Med;77(3).

Mussig K. Kunle A, Sauberlich AL, Weinert

C, et al. Thyroid peroxidase antibody positivity is associated with symptomatic distress in patients with Hashimoto's thyroiditis. 2012 Brain Behav Immun;26(4):559-63.

Paparodis R, Imam S, Todorova-Koteva K, et al. Hashimoto's Thyroiditis Pathology and Risk for Thyroid Cancer. 2014 Thyroid 1; 24(7):1107-1114.

Pearce EN. National trends in iodine nutrition: is everyone getting enough? 2007 Thyroid;17(9): 823-7.

Rio Frio T, et al. DICER1 mutations in familial multinodular goiter with and without ovarian Sertoli-Leydig cell tumors. 2011 JAMA;305:68-77.

Roduit C et al. Prenatal Animal Contact and Gene Expression of Innate Immunity Receptors at Birth Are Associated with Atopic Dermatitis. 2011 J Allergy Clin Immunol;127(91).

Rosenfeld L. Discovery and early uses of iodine. 2000 J Chem Educ;77:984-987.

Sawin, CT. Hakaru Hashimoto (1881-1934) and his disease. 2001 The Endocrinologist;11(2):73-76.

Sawin, CT. The heritage of Dr. Hakaru Hashimoto (1881-1934). 2002 Endocrine;49(4):399-403.

Tagoe CE, Zezon A, Khattri S, Castellanos P. Rheumatic manifestations of euthyroid, anti-thyroid antibody-positive patients. 2013 Rheumatol Int;33(7):1745-52.

Volpé R. The Life of Dr. Hakaru Hashimoto. 1989 Autoimmunity;3(4):243-245.

Von Ehrenstein OS, et al. Reduced Risk of Hay Fever and Asthma Among Children of Farmers. 2002 Clin Exp Allergy:30(2):187-93.

Waite KJ. Blackley and the Development of Hay Fever as a Disease of Civilization in the Nineteenth Century. 1995 Medical History;39(2):186-196.

Zimmerman MD. Research on iodine deficiency and goiter in the 19th and early 20th centuries. 2008 J Nutr;138(11):2060-3.

Chapter 3

Abalovich, M., Mitelberg, L., Allami, C., et al. Subclinical hypothyroidism and thyroid autoimmunity in women with infertility. 2007 Gynecol Endocrinol 23(5):279-283.

Brearley KD, Spiers AS. Autoimmune disease of the thyroid and colon, with a report of a case of chronic ulcerative colitis in association with Hashimoto's disease and penicillin allergy. 1962 Med J Aust;49(1):789-95.

Carp HJA, Selmi C, Shoenfeld Y. The autoimmune bases of infertility and pregnancy loss. 2012 J Autoimmun 38(2-3):J266-J274.

Caturegli P, De Remigis A, Rose NR. Hashimoto thyroiditis: Clinical and diagnostic criteria. 2014 Autoimmun Rev; 13:391-397.

de Vivo a, et al. Thyroid function in women found to have early pregnancy loss. 2010 Thyroid:20(6):633-637.

Degirmenci PB, et al. Allergic rhinitis and its relationship with autoimmune thyroid diseases. 2015 Am J Rhinol Allergy;29(4):357-61.

Desailloud R, Hober D. Viruses and thyroiditis: an update. Virol J. 2009;6:5.

G. E. Krassas, K. Poppe, and D. Glinoer, Thyroid function and human reproductive health. 2010 Endocr Rev;31(5):702-755.

Twig G, Shina A, Amital H, Shoenfeld Y. Pathogenesis of infertility and recurrent pregnancy loss in thyroid autoimmunity. 2012 J Autoimmun;38(2-3):J275-J281.

Hall R, Stanbury JB. Familial studies of autoimmune thyroiditis. 1967 Am J Clin Exp Immunol;2(Suppl):719-25.

Hollowell JG, Staehling NW, Flanders WD, et al. Serum TSH, T(4), and thyroid antibodies in the United States population (1988 to 1994): National Health and Nutrition Examination Survey (NHANES III). 2002 J Clin Endocrinol Metab;87(2):489-499.

Jabrocka-Hybel A, Shalniak A, Piatkowski J, Pach D, Hubalewska-Dydejczyk A. How far are we from understanding the genetic basis of Hashimoto's thyroiditis? 2013 Int Rev Immunol;32(3):337-54.

Poppe K, Glinoer D, van Steirteghem A, et al., Thyroid dysfunction and autoimmunity infertile women. 2002 Thyroid;12(11):997-1001.

Lee HJ, Li CW, Hammerstad SS, Stefan M, Tomer Y. Immunogenetics of autoimmune thyroid diseases: A comprehensive review. 2015 J Autoimmun 64:82-90.

McLeod DS, Cooper DS. The incidence and prevalence of thyroid autoimmunity. 2012 Endocrine; 42(2):252-265.

McLeod DS, Caturegli P, Cooper DS, Matos PG, Hutfless S. Variation in rates of autoimmune thyroid disease by race/ethnicity in US military personnel. 2014 JAMA;311(15):1563-5.

Minegaki Y, Higashida Y, Ogawa M, Miyachi Y, Fujii H, Kabashima K. Drug-induced hypersensitivity syndrome complicated with concurrent fulminant type 1 diabetes mellitus and Hashimoto's thyroiditis. 2013 Int J Dermatol;52(3):355-7.

Caturegli P, De Remigis A, Rose NR. Hashimoto thyroiditis: Clinical and diagnostic criteria. 2014 Autoimmun Rev;13:391-397.

Pyzik A, Grywalska E, Matyjaszek-Matuszek B, Rolinski J. Immune Disorders in Hashimoto's Thyroiditis: What Do We Know So Far? 2015 J Immunol Res;2015:979167.

Rajic B, Arapovic J, Raguz K, Boskovic M, Babic SM, Maslac S. Eradiaction of Blastocystis hominis prevents the development of symptomatic Hashimoto's thyroiditis: a case report. 2015 J Infect Dev Ctries;9(7):788-91.

Tomer Y, Davies TF. Searching for the autoimmune thyroid disease susceptibility genes: from gene mapping to gene function. 2003 Endocr Rev;24:694-717.

Villanueva R, Greenberg DA, Davies TF, Tomer Y. Sibling recurrence risk in autoimmune thyroid disease. 2003 Thyroid;13:761-4.

Chapter 4

Agarwal K, Jones DE, Daly AK, James OF, Vaidya B, Pearce S, et al. CTLA-4 gene polymorphism confers susceptibility to primary biliary cirrhosis. 2000 Int. J. Hepatol;32:538-41.

Agmon-Levin N, Zafrir Y, Kivity S, Balofsky A, Amital H, Shoenfeld Y. Chronic fatigue syndrome and fibromyalgia following immunization with the hepatitis B vaccine: another angle of the 'autoimmune (auto-inflammatory) syndrome induced by adjuvants' (ASIA). 2014 Immunol Res;60(2-3):376-83.

Ahmad J, Tagoe CE. Fibromyalgia and chronic widespread pain in autoimmune thyroid disease. 2014 Clin Rheumatol;33(7):885-91.

Anaya JM. The Autoimmune tautology. 2010 Arthritis Res Ther;12(6):147.

Baethge BA, Levine SN, Wolf RE. Antibodies to nuclear antigens in Graves' disease. 1988 J Clin Endocrinol Metab;66(3):485-8.

Baldini E, Odorisio T, Sorrenti S, Catania A, Tartaglia F et al. Vitiligo and Autoimmune Thyroid Disorders. 2017 Front Endocrinol;8:290.

Ban Y, Tozaki T, Tobe T, Ban Y, Jacobson EM, Concepcion ES, et al. The regulatory T cell gene FOXP3 and genetic susceptibility to thyroid autoimmunity: an association analysis in Caucasian and Japanese cohorts. 2007 J Autoimmun;28:201-7

Blitshteyn S. Autoimmune markers and autoimmune disorders in patients with postural tachycardia syndrome (POTS). 2015 Lupus;24(13):1364-9.

Boelaert K, Newby PR, Simmonds MJ, Holder RL et al. Prevalence and relative risk of other autoimmune diseases in subjects with autoimmune thyroid disease. 2010 Am J Med;123(2):183.e1-9.

Bossowski A, Czarnocka B, Bardadin K, Stasiak-Barmuta A, Urban M, Dadan J, Ratomski K. Identification of apoptotic proteins in thyroid gland from patients with Graves' disease and Hashimoto's thyroiditis. 2008 Autoimmunity;41(2):163-73.

Bottini N, Musumeci L, Alonso A, Rahmouni S, Nika K, Rostamkhani M, et al. A functional variant of lymphoid tyrosine phosphatase is associated with type I diabetes. 2004 Nature Genet;36:337-8.

Brahmkshatriya PP, Mehta AA, Saboo BD, Goyal RK. Characteristics and Prevalence of Latent Autoimmune Diabetes in Adulthood (LADA). 2012 ISRN Pharmacol;2012/580202.

Cardenas-Roldan J, Rojas-Villarraga A, Anaya J-M. How do autoimmune diseases cluster in families? A systematic review and meta-analysis. 2013 BMC Med;11:73.

Carlton VE, Hu X, Chokkalingam AP, Schrodi SJ, Brandon R, Alexander HC, et al. PTPN22 genetic variation: evidence for multiple variants associated with rheumatoid arthritis. 2005 Am J Hum Genet;77:567-81.

Chistiakov DA, Chistiakov AP. Is FCRL3 a new general autoimmunity gene? 2007 Hum immunol;68:375-83.

Cojocaru M, Mihaela I, Silosi I. Multiple Autoimmune Disease. 2010 Maedica (Buchar); 5(2):132-134.

Djilali-Saiah I, Schmitz J, Harfouch-Hammoud E, Mougenot JF, Bach JF, Caillat-Zucman S. CTLA-4 gene polymorphism is associated with predisposition to coeliac disease. 1988 Gut;43:187-9.

Downie-Doyle S, Bayat N, Rischmueller M, Lester S. Influence of CTLA4 haplotypes on susceptibility and some extraglandular manifestations in primary Sjogren's syndrome. 2006 Arthritis Rheum;54:2434-40.

Franco JS, Amaya-Amaya J, Molano-Gonzalez N, et al. Autoimmune thyroid disease in Colombian patients with systemic lupus erythematosus. 2015 Clin Endocrinol (Oxf);83(6):943-50.

Harjutsalo V, Reunanen A, Tuomilehto J. Differential Transmission of Type 1 Diabetes from Diabetic Fathers and Mothers To Their Offspring. 2006 Diabetes;55(5):1517-1524.

Hemminki K, Li X, Sundquist J, Sundquist K. Familial associations of rheumatoid arthritis with autoimmune diseases. 2009 Arthritis Rheum;60(3):661-8.

Huang D, Liu L, Noren K, Xia SQ, Trifunovic J, Pirskanen R, et al. Genetic association of Ctla-4 to myasthenia gravis with thymoma. 1998 J Neuroimmunol;88:192-8.

Inamo Y, Harada K. Antinuclear antibody positivity in pediatric patients with autoimmune thyroid disease.1997 J Rheumatol;24(3):576-8.

Jenkins RC, Weetman AP. Disease associations with autoimmune thyroid disease. 2002 Thyroid;12:977-88.

Katoh H, Zheng P, Liu Y. FOXP3: genetic and epigenetic implications for autoimmunity. 2013 J Autoimmun;41:72-8.

Kyogoku C, Langefeld CD, Ortmann WA, Lee A, Selby S, Carlton VE, et al. Genetic association of the R620W polymorphism of protein tyrosine phosphatase PTPN22 with human SLE. 2004 Human Genet;75:504-7.

Lee YH, Harley JB, Nath SK. CTLA-4 polymorphisms and systemic lupus erythematosus (SLE): a meta-analysis. 2005 Human Genet;116:361-7.

Lee, HJ, Li CW, Hammerstad SS, Stefan M, Tomer Y. Immunogenetics of Autoimmune Thyroid Diseases: A Comprehensive Review. 2015 J Autoimmun;64: 82-90.

Li CW, Concepcion E, Tomer Y. Dissecting the role of the FOXP3 gene in the joint genetic susceptibility to autoimmune thyroiditis and diabetes: a genetic and functional analysis. 2015 Gene;556:142-8.

Li H, Yu X, Liles C, Khan M, et al. Autoimmune basis for postural tachycardia syndrome. 2014 J Am Heart Assoc;26;3(1).

Li K, Zhao M, Hou S, Du L, Kijlstra A, Yang P. Association between polymorphisms of FCRL3, a non-HLA gene, and Behcet's disease in a Chinese population with ophthalmic manifestations. 2008 Mol Vis;14:2136-42.

Maes M, Leunis JC. Attenuation of autoimmune responses to oxidative specific epitopes, but not nitroso-adducts, is associated with a better clinical outcome in Myalgic Encephalomyelitis/chronic fatigue syndrome. 2014 Neuro Endocrunol Lett;35(7):577-85.

Morris G, Berk M, Galecki P, Maes M. The emerging role of autoimmunity in myalgic encephalomyelitis/chronic fatigue syndrome (ME/cfs). 2014 Mol Neurobiol;49(2):741-56.

Pan XF, Gu JQ, Shan ZY. The prevalance of thyroid autoimmunity in patients with urticaria: a systematic review and meta-analysis. 2015 Endocrine;48(3):804-10.

Shah SA, Peppercorn MA, Pallotta JA. Autoimmune (Hashimoto's) thyroiditis associated with Crohn's Disease. 1998 J Clin Gastroenterol;26(2):117-20.

Sloka JS, Phillips P, Stefanelli M, Joyce C. Co-occurrence of autoimmune thyroid disease. 2005 J Autoimmune Dis;2:9.

Song GG, Lee YH. The CTLA-4 and MCP-1 polymorphisms and susceptibility to systemic sclerosis: a meta-analysis. 2013 Immunol Invest;42:481-92.

Suk JH, Lee JH, Kim JM. Association between thyroid autoimmunity and fibromyalgia. 2012 Exp Clin Endocrinol Diabetes:120(7):401-4.

Svejgaard A, Platz P, Ryder LP. HLA and disease 1982--a survey. 1983 Immunol Rev;70:193-218.

Todd JA, Acha-Orbea H, Bell JI, Chao N, Fronek Z, Jacob CO, et al. A molecular basis for MHC class II--associated autoimmunity. 1988 Science;240:1003-9.

Tomer Y, Menconi F. Type 1 Diabetes and Autoimmune Thyroiditis: The Genetic Connection. 2009 Thyroid;19(2):99-102.

Vaidya B, Imrie H, Geatch DR, Perros P, Ball SG, Baylis PH, et al. Association analysis of the cytotoxic T lymphocyte antigen-4 (CTLA-4) and autoimmune regulator-1 (AIRE-1) genes in sporadic autoimmune Addison's disease. 2000 J Clin Endocrinol Metab;85:688-91.

Velaga MR, Wilson V, Jennings CE, Owen CJ, Herington S, Donaldson PT, et al. The codon 620 tryptophan allele of the lymphoid tyrosine phosphatase (LYP) gene is a major determinant of Graves' disease. 2004 J Clin Endocrinol Metab;89:5862-5.

Villano MJ, Huber AK, Greenberg DA, Golden BK, Concepcion E, Tomer Y. Autoimmune thyroiditis and diabetes: dissecting the joint genetic susceptibility in a large cohort of multiplex families. 2009 J Clin Endocrinol Metab;94:1458-66.

Wang X, Yu T, Yan Q, Wang W, Meng N, Li X, et al. Significant Association Between Fc ReceptorLike 3 Polymorphisms (-1901A>G and -658C>T) and Neuromyelitis Optica (NMO) Susceptibility in the Chinese Population. 2015 Mol Neurobiol.

Yuan M, Wei L, Zhou R, Bai Q, Wei Y, Zhang W, et al. Four FCRL3 Gene Polymorphisms (FCRL3_3, _5, _6, _8) Confer Susceptibility to Multiple Sclerosis: Results from a Case-Control Study. 2015 Mol Neurobiol.

Chapter 5

American Academy of Anti-Aging Medicine (A4M). White Paper Guidance for Physicians on Hormone Replacement Therapy (HRT). 27 April 2007 [updated 22 May 2007; Cited 17 August 2018]. Available from: https://jeffreydachmd.com/wp-content/uploads/2013/03/White-Paper-Guidance-for-Physicians-on-Hormone-Replacement-Therapy-2007-A4M.pdf

Austen FK, Rubini ME, Meroney WH, Wolff J. Salicylates and thyroid function. I. Depression of thyroid function. 1958 J Clin Invest;37:1131-114.

Azizi F, Mannix JE, Howard D, Nelson RA. Effect of winter sleep on pituitary-thyroid axis in American black bear. 1979 Am J Physiol;237(3): E227-30.

Azizi F, Vagenakis AG, Portnay GI, et al: Thyroxine transport and metabolism in methadone and heroin addicts. 1974 Ann Intern Med;80:194-199.

Baloch Z, Carayon P, Conte-Devoix B, Demers LM, Feldt-Rasmussen U, Henry JF. Et al. Laboratory support for the diagnosis and monitoring of thyroid disease. 2003 Thyroid;13:3-126.

Barchetta I, Baroni MG, Leonetti F, De Bernardinis M, Bertoccini L, Fontana M, Mazzei E, Fraioli A, Cavallo MG. TSH levels are associated with vitamin D status and seasonaility in an adult population of euthyroid adults. 2015 Clin Exp Med;15(3):389-96.

Baskin et al. 2002 Endocrine Practice;8:457.

Baskin HJ, Cobin RH, Duick DS, Gharib H, Guttler RB, Kaplan MM, Segal RL. American Association of Clinical Endocrinologists Medical Guidelines for Clinical Practice for the Evaluation and Treatment of Hyperthyroidism and Hypothyroidism. AACE Thyroid Task Force. 2002 Endocrine Practice;8(6):457-69.

Bianco AC. Cracking the code for thyroid hormone signaling. 2013 Trans Am Clin Climatol Assoc;124:24-35.

Bohinc BN, Michelotti G, Pang H, Suzuki A, Guy CD, Piercy D, Jruger L, Swiderska-Syn M, Machado M, Pereira T, Zavacki AM, Abdelmalek M, Diehl AM. Repair-related activation of hedgehog signaling in stromal cells promotes intrahepatic hypothyroidism. 2014 Endocrinology; 155(11): 4591-601.

Bray GA, Hildreth S. Effect of propylthiouracil and methimazole on the oxygen consumption of hypothyroid rats receiving thyroxine or triiodothyronine. 1967 Endocrinology;81:1018.

Burger A, Dinichert D, Nicod P, et al. Effects of amiodarone on serum triiodothyronine, reverse triiodothyronine, thyroxine and thyrotropin. 1976 J Clin Invest 58:255-259.

Cashin-Hemphill L, Spencer CA, Nocoloff JT, et al. Alterations in serum thyroid hormonal indices with colestipol-niacin therapy. 1987 Ann Intern Med 107:324-329.

Chopra IJ, Solomon DH, Chopra U, Wu SY,

Fisher DA, Nakamura Y. Pathways of metabolism of thyroid hormones. 1978 Recent Prog Horm Res 34:521.

Chopra IJ, Williams DE, Orgiazzi J, Solomon DH. Opposite effects of dexamethasone on serum concentrations of 3,3',5'-triiodothyronine (reverse T3) and 3,3',5-triiodothyronine (T3). 1975 J Clin Endocrinol Metab;41:911-920.

Christensen LK. Thyroxine-releasing effect of salicylate and of 2,4-dinitrophenol. 1959 Nature 183:1189-1190.

David S. Cooper, Gerard M. Doherty, Bryan R. Haugen, Richard T. Kloos, Stephanie L. Lee, Susan J. Mandel, Ernest L. Mazzaferri, Bryan McIver, Furio Pacini, Martin Schlumberger, Steven I. Sherman, David L. Steward, and R. Michael Tuttle. Revised American Thyroid Association Management Guidelines for Patients with Thyroid Nodules and Differentiated Thyroid Cancer. 2009 Thyroid;19(11).

Dong BJ. How medications affect thyroid function. 2000 West J Med;172(2):102-106.

Dowling JT, Frienkel N, Ingbar SH: The effect of estrogens upon the peripheral metabolism of thyroxine. 1974 J Clin Invest 39:1119-1130.

Draper MW, Flowers, DE, Neild JA, Huster WJ, Zerbe RL: Antiestrogenic properties of raloxifene. 1995 Pharmacology 50:209-17.

Duick DS, Warren DW, Nicoloff JT, et al: Effect of a single dose of dexamethasone on the concentration of serum triiodothyronine in man. 1974 J Clin Endocrinol Metab 39:1151-1154.

Gabrilove JL, Alvarez AA, Soffer LJ: Effect of acetazoleamide (Diamox) on thyroid function. 1958 J Appl Physiol;13:491.

Haugen B, et al. American Thyroid Association Management Guidelines for Adult Patients with Thyroid Nodules and Differentiated Thyroid Cancer: The American Thyroid Association Guidelines Task Force on Thyroid Nodules. 2015 Thyroid;(26)1.

Hershman JM, Jones CM, Bailey AL. Reciprocal changes in serum thyrotropin and free thyroxine produced by heparin. 1972 J Clin Endocrinol Metab;34:574.

Hollowell JG, Staehling NW, Flanders WD, Hannon WH, Gunter EW, Spencer CA, Braverman LE. Serum TSH, T4, and Thyroid Antibodies in the United States Population (1988 to 1994): National Health and Nutrition Examination Survey (NHANES III). 2002 J Clin Endocrinol Metab;87(2).

Krieger DT, Moses A, Ziffer H, Gabrilove JL, Soffer LJ: Effect of acetazoleamide on thyroid metabolism. 1959 Am J Physiol;196:291.

Larsen PR. Salicylate-induced increases in free triiodothyronine in human serum: Evidence of inhibition of triiodothyronine binding to thyroxine-binding globulin and thyroxine-binding prealbumin. 1972 J Clin Invest;51:1125-1134.

Levy SB, Leonard WR, Tarsakaia LA, Klimova TM, Fedorova VI, Baltakhinova ME, Krivoshapkin VG, Snodgrass JJ. Seasonal and socioeconomic influences on thyroid function among the Yakut (Sakha) of Eastern Siberia. 2013 Am J Hum Biol;25(6):814-20.

McKerron CG, Scott RL, Asper SP, Levy RI: Effects of clofibrate (Atromid S) on the thyroxine-binding capacity of thyroxine-binding globulin and free thyroxine. 1969 J Clin Endocrinol Metab;29:957-961.

Morley JE, Shafer RB, Elson MK, et al: Amphetamine-induced hyperthyroxinemia. 1980 Ann Int Med;93:707-709.

Moura Neto A, Parisi MC, Tambascia MA, Alegre SM, Pavin EJ, Zantut-Wittmann DE. The influence of body mass index and low-grade systemic inflammation on thyroid hormone abnormalities in patients with diabetes. 2013 Endocr J;60(7):877-84.

Northcutt RC, Stiel MN, Nollifield JW, Stant EG Jr.: The influence of cholestyramine on thyroxine absorption. 1969 JAMA;208:1857-1861.

Price A. Obel O. Cresswell J. Catch I. Rutter S. Barik S. Heller SR. Weetman AP. Comparison of thyroid function in pregnant and non-pregnant Asian and western Caucasian women. 2001 Clin Chim Acta;308:91-98.

Raitiere MN. Clinical evidence for thyroid dysfunction in patients with seasonal affective disorder. 1992 Psychoneuroendocrinology;17(2-3): 231-41.

Razvi S, Shakoor A, Vanderpump M, Weaver J.U, Pearce S. The Influence of Age on the Relationship Between Subclinical Hypothyroidism and Ischemic Heart Disease: A Metaanalysis. 2008 J Clin Endocrinol Metab;93(8):2998-3007.

Rootwelt K, Ganes T, Johannessen SI: Effect of carbamazapine, phenytoin and phenobarbitone on serum levels of thyroid hormones and thyrotropin in humans. 1978 Scand J Clin Lab Invest;38:731-736.

Salvatore D, Davies TF, Schlumberger MJ, Hay ID, Larsen PR. Thyroid physiology and diagnostic evaluation of patients with thyroid disorders. In: Melmed S, et al, eds. Williams Textbook of Endocrinology. 13th ed. Philadelphia: Elsevier; 2016.

Sander M, Rocker L. Influence of marathon running on thyroid hormones. 1988 Int J Sports Med;9(2):123-6.

Schatz D, Sheppard R, Steiner G, et al. Influence of heparin on serum free thyroxine. 1969 J Clin Endocrinol Metab;29:1015-1022.

Skinner NS, Hayes RL, Hill SR. Studies on the use of chlorpropamide in patients with diabetes mellitus. 1959 Ann NY Acad Sci;74:83.

Smals AG, Kloppenborg PW, Hoefnagesl WH, Drayer JM. Pituitary-thyroid function in spirolactone treated hypertensive women. 1979 Acta Endocrinol;90:577-584.

Stagnaro-Green A, Abalovich M, Alexander E, Azizi F, Mestman J, Negro R, Nixon A, Pearce EN, Soldin OP, Sullivan S, Wiersinga W. Guidelines of the American Thyroid Association for the Diagnosis and Management of Thyroid Disease During Pregnancy and Postpartum. 2011 Thyroid;21(10):1081-1125.

Stockigt JR, Lim CF, Barlow JW, et al: Interaction of furosemide with serum thyroxine-binding sites: In vivo and in vitro studies and comparison with other inhibitors. 1985 J Clin Endocrinol Metab;60:1025-1031.

Sviridonova MA, Fadeyev VV, Sych YP, Melnichenko GA. Clinical Significance of TSH Circadian Variability in Patients with Hypothyroidism. 2013 Endocr Res;38.

Tabachnick M, Hao YL, Korcek L: Effect of oleate, diphenylhydantoin, and heparin on the binding of 125I-thyroxine to purified thyroxine-binding globulin. 1973 J Clin Endocrinol Metab;36:392-394.

Tomasi TE, Hellgren EC, Tucker TJ. Thyroid hormone concentrations in black bears (Ursus americanus): hibernation and pregnancy effects. 1998 Gen Comp Endocrinol;109(2):192-9.

Vadivello T, Donnan PT, Murphy MJ, Leese GP. Age- and Gender-Specific TSH Reference Intervals in People With No Obvious Thyroid Disease in Tayside, Scotland: The Thyroid Epidemiology, Audit, and Research Study (TEARS). 2013 J Clin Endocrin Metab;98(3).

Weiss RE, Refetoff S. Thyroid function testing. In: Jameson JL, De Groot LJ, de Kretser DM, et al, eds. Endocrinology: Adult and Pediatric. 7th ed. Philadelphia: Elsevier; 2016.

Wolff J, Austen FK. Salicylates and thyroid function. II. The effect on the thyroid-pituitary interrelation. 1958 J Clin Invest;37:1144-1165.

Figure 5.1 and all tables (except Table 12.1) source: Brittany Henderson

Table 12.1: Allison Futterman

Chapter 6

Duick DS, Levine RA, Lupo MA, eds. Thyroid and Parathyroid Ultrasound and Ultrasound-Guided FNA. 4th Ed. New York: Springer International Publishing; 2018.

Chapter 7

Cibas ES, Ali SZ. NCI Thyroid FNA State of the Science Conference. The Bethesda System for Reporting Thyroid Cytopathology. 2009 Am J Clin Pathol;132(5):658-65.

Haugen BR, Alexander EK, Bible KC, Doherty GM, Mandel SJ, Nikiforov YE, Pancini F, Randolph GW, Sawka AM, Schlumberger M, Schuff KG, Sherman SI, Sosa JA, Steward DL, Tuttle RM, Wartofsky L. 2015 American Thyroid Association Management Guidelines for Adult Patients with Thyroid Nodules and Differentiated Thyroid Cancer. 2016 Thyroid; 26(1):1-133.

Table 7.1 information adapted from Cibas ES, Ali SZ. NCI Thyroid FNA State of the Science Conference. The Bethesda System for Reporting Thyroid Cytopathology. 2009 Am J Clin Pathol;132(5):658-65.

Chapter 8

American Thyroid Association, Endocrine Society, American Association of Clinical Endocrinologists. Joint statement on the U.S. Food and Drug Administration's decision regarding bioequivalence of levothyroxine sodium. 2004 Thyroid;14:486.

Brown T. The 10 Most-Prescribed and Top-Selling Medications [Internet]. WebMD. WebMD; 2015 [Cited 2018 Aug 17]. Available from: https://www.webmd.com/drug-medication/news/20150508/most-prescribed-top-selling-drugs

Center for Drug Evaluation and Research. Drug Applications for Over-the-Counter (OTC) Drugs [Internet]. U S Food and Drug Administration Home Page. Center for Biologics Evaluation and Research; [Cited 2018 Aug 17]. Available from: https://www.fda.gov/Drugs/DevelopmentApprovalProcess/HowDrugsareDevelopedandApproved/ApprovalApplications/Over-the-CounterDrugs/default.htm

Center for Drug Evaluation and Research. How Drugs are Developed and Approved [Internet]. US Food and Drug Administration Home Page. Center for Biologics Evaluation and Research; [Cited 2018 Aug 17]. Available from: https://www.fda.gov/Drugs/DevelopmentApprovalProcess/HowDrugsareDevelopedandApproved/

Office of the Commissioner. What We Do. US Food and Drug Administration Home Page. Center for Biologics Evaluation and Research; [Cited 2018 Aug 17]. Available from: https://www.fda.gov/AboutFDA/WhatWeDo/

Chapter 9

Abdollahi-Roodsaz S, Abramson SB, Scher JU. The metabolic role of the cut micro bio dad health and rheumatic disease Colin mechanisms and interventions. 2016 Nat Rev Rheumatol;12(8):446-55.

Alipour B, Homayouni-Rad A, Vaghef-Mehrabany E, Sharif SK, Vaghef-Mehrabany L, Asghari-Jafarabadi M, Nakhjavani MR, Mohtadi-Nia J. effects of Lactobacillus casei supplementation a disease activity and inflammatory cytokines in rheumatoid arthritis patients: a randomized double-blind clinical trial. 2014 Int J Rheum Dis;17(5):519-27.

Belkaid Y, Hand TW. Role of the microbiota in immunity and inflammation. 2014 Cell;157(1):121-41.

Bernstein AM, Song M, Zhang X, Pan A, Wang M, Fuchs CS, Le N, Chan AT, Willett WC, Ogino S, Giovannucci EL, Wu K. Processed and Unprocessed Red Meat and Risk of Colorectal cancer: Analysis by Tumor Location and Modification by Time. 2015 PLoS One;10(8):e0135959.

L.D. KZRD. What is BVO and why is it in my soda? [Internet]. Mayo Clinic. Mayo Foundation for Medical Education and Research; 2016 [Cited 2018 Aug 17]. Available from: https://www.mayoclinic.org/healthy-lifestyle/nutrition-and-healthy-eating/expert-answers/bvo/faq-20058236

Ciccia F, Guggino G, Rizzo A, Alessandro R, Luchetti M, Milling S, Saieva L, Cypers H, Stampone T, Benedetto P, Gabrielli A,

Fasano A, Elewaut D, Triolo G. Dysbiosis and zonulin upregulation alter gut.epithelial and vascular barriers in patients with ankylosing spondylitis. 2017 Ann Rheum Dis;76(6):1123-1132.

Citi S. Intestinal barriers protect against disease. 2018 Science;359(6380):1097-98.

Cordain L, Toohey L, Smith MJ, Hickey MS. Modulation of the main function by dietary lectins in rheumatoid arthritis. 2000 Br J Nutr;83(03):207-217.

De Punder K, Pruimboom L. the dietary intake of wheat and other cereal grains and their role in inflammation. 2013 Nutrients;12:5(3):771-87.

Ming L, Wenjuan G, Jingjing M, Yun Z, Xingfu L. Early-stage lupus nephritis treated with NAC: a report of two cases. 2015 Exp Ther Med;10(2):689-692.

Center for Food Safety and Applied Nutrition. Food Additives & Ingredients - Food Additive Status List [Internet]. US Food and Drug Administration Home Page. Center for Biologics Evaluation and Research; [Cited 2018 Aug 17]. Available from: https://www.fda.gov/Food/IngredientsPackagingLabeling/FoodAdditivesIngredients/ucm091048.htm

https://www.fda.gov/food/labelingnutrition/ucm275409.htm

Frankenfeld CL, Sikaroodi M, Lamb E, Shoemaker S, Gillevet PM. High intensity sweetener consumption and gut microbiome content in predicted gene function in a cross-sectional study of adults in the United States. 2015 Ann Epidemiolt;25(10):736-42.e4.

Gao Y, Bielohuby M, Fleming T, et al. Dietary sugars, not lipids, drive hypothalamic inflammation. 2017 Mol Metab;6(8):897-908.

Haghikia A, et al. Dietary fatty acids directly impact CNS autoimmunity via the small intestines. 2015 Immunity;43(4):817-29.

Hernandez AL, Kitz A, Wu C, Lowther DE et al. Sodiu, chloride inhibits the suppressive function of FOXP3+ regulatory T cells. 2015 J Clin Invest;125(11):4212-22.

Hewison M. Vitamin D and immune function: an overview. 2012 Proc Nutr Soc;71(1):50-61.

Ho S, Woodford K, Kukuljan S, Pal S. Comparative effects of A1 versus A2 beta-casein on gastrointestinal measures: a blinded randomised cross-over pilot study. 2014 Eur J Nutr; 68(9): 994-1000.

Hu S, Rayman M. Multiple nutritional factors and the risk of Hashimoto's thyroiditis. 2017 Thyroid;27(5).

Jameel F, Phang M, Wood LG, Garg ML. Acute effects of feeding fructose, glucose and sucrose on blood lipid levels and systemic inflammation. 2014 Lipids Health Dis;13:195.

Johnson D, O'Connor S. Genetically Modified Foods: What Is Grown and Eaten in the U.S [Internet]. Time; 30 Apr 2018 [Cited 17 Aug 2018]. Available from: http://time.com/3840073/gmo-food-charts/

Lai ZW et al. N-acetylcysteine reduces disease activity by blocking mammalian target of rapamycin in T cells from systemic lupus erythematosus patients: a randomized, double-blind, placebo-controlled trial. 2012 Arthritis Rhuem; 64(9):689-692.

Liontiris M, Mazokopakis E. a concise review of Hasheem it is very dangerous in the importance of iodine, selenium, vitamin D and gluten. 2017 Hell J Nucl Med;20(1):51-56.

Mesnage R, Agapito-Tenfan SZ, Vilperte V, Renney G et al. An integrated muli-omics analysis of the NK603 Roundup-tolerant GM maize reveals metabolism disturbances caused by the transformation process. 2016 Sci Rep;6:37855.

Metso S, Hyytua-Ilmonen H, Kaukinen K, et al. Gluten free diet and autoimmune peritonitis in patients with celiac disease. A prospective controlled study. 2012 Scand J Gastroenterol;47(1):43-8.

Moreno-Navarrete JM, Sabater M, Ortega F,

Ricart W, Fernandez-Real, JM. Circulating zonulin, a marker of intestinal permeability, it is increased in association with obesity associated insulin resistance. 2012 PLoS One;7(5):e37160.

NAC decreases disease activity by blocking mTOR in T cells in lupus patients. 2012 Arthritis Rhuem;64(9):689-692.

Naiyer AJ, Shah J, Hernandez L, Kim SY et al. Tissue transglutaminase antibodies in individuals with celiac disease bind to thyroid follicles and extra cellular matrix and make contribute to thyroid dysfunction. 2008 Thyroid;18(11):1171-8.

Otto MA. AACE: Artificial sweeteners tentatively linked to Hashimoto's thyroiditis [Internet]. Clinical Endocrinology News; 21 May 2015 [Cited 2018 Aug 17]. Available from: https://www.mdedge.com/clinicalendocrinologynews/article/99841/pituitary-thyroid-adrenal-disorders/aace-artificial

Palmnas MS, Cowan TE, Bomhof MR, Su J, Reimer RA, Vogel HJ, Hittel DS, Shearer J. Low-dose aspartame consumption differentially affects gut microbiota-host metabolic interactions in the diet-induced obese rate. 2014 PLoS One;9(10):e109841.

Peckham S, Lowery D, Spencer S. Are fluoride levels in drinking water associated with hypothyroidism prevalence in England? A large observational study of GP practice data and fluoride levels in drinking water. 2015 J Epidemiol Community Health;69(7):619-24.

Perez-Abud R, Rodriguez-Gomez I, Villarejo AB, Moreno JM et al. Salt Sensitvity in experimental thyroid disorders in rats. 2011 Am J Physiol Endocrinol Metab;301(2):E281-7.

Suaini NHA, Zhang Y, Vuillermin PJ, Allen KJ, Harrison LC. I mean modulation by vitamin D and its relevance to food allergy. 2015 Nutrients;7(8):6088-6108.

Suez J, et al. Artificial sweeteners induce glucose intolerance by altering the gut microbiota. 2014 Nature;514(7521):181-6.

Sultana R, McBain AJ, O'Neill CA. Strain-Dependent Augmentation of Tight-Junction barrier function in human primary epidermal keratinocytes by Lactobacillus and Bifidobacterium Lysates. 2013 Appl Environ Microbiol;79(16):4887-94.

Turnbaugh PJ et al. Core microbiome in obese and lean twins: Missouri Adolescent Female Twin study. 2009 Nature;457:480-484.

Ul Haq MR, Kapila R, Sharma R, Saliganti V, Kapila S. Comparative evaluation of cow B-casein variants (A1/A2) consumption on Th2-mediated inflammatory response in mouse gut. 2014 Eur J Nutr;53(4):1039-49.

Ulven SM, Holven KB. Comparison of bio-availability of krill oil versus fish oil and health effect. 2015 Vascular Health and Risk Management;11:511-524.

Vieira SM, Hiltensperger M et al. Translocation of a gut pathobiont Drive auto-immunity in mice and humans. 2018 Science;359(6380):1156-61.

Vighi, G., Marcucci, F., Sensi, L., Di Cara, G., & Frati, F. (2008). Allergy and the gastrointestinal system. Clinical and Experimental Immunology, 153(Suppl 1), 3–6.

Yang Q, Zhang Z, Gregg EW, Flanders WD, Merritt R, Hu FB. Added Sugar Intake and Cardiovascular Diseases Mortality Among US Adults. 2014 JAMA Intern Med;174(4):516-524

Zhang M, Yang X-J. Effects of a high fat diet on intestinal microbiota and gastrointestinal diseases. 2016 World J Gastroenterol;22(40):8905-8909.`

Chapter 10

Abbas AM, Sakr HF. Effect of magnesium sulfate and thyroxine and inflammatory markers in a rat model of hypothyroidism. 2016 Can J Physiol Pharmacol;94(4):426-32.

Benvenga S, Vigo MT, Metro D, Granese R, Vita R, Le Donne M. Type of Fish consumed and thyroid autoimmunity in pregnancy and postpartum. 2016 Endocrine;52(1):120-9.

Bozkurt NC, Karbek B, Ucan B, Sahin M, Cakal E, Ozbek M, Delibasi T. The association between severity of vitamin D deficiency and Hashimoto's thyroiditis. 2013 Endocr Pract;19(3):479-84.

Bright JJ. Curcumin and autoimmune disease. Adv Exp Med Biol. 2007; 595:425-51.

Calder PC. Omega-3 polyunsaturated fatty acids and inflammatory processes: nutrition or pharmacology? 2013 Br J Clin Pharmacol;75(3):645-62.

Costantini A, Pala MI. Thiamine and Hashimoto's thyroiditis: a report of three cases. 2014 J Altern Complement Med;20(3):208-11.

D'Ambrosio DN, Clugston RD, Blaner WS. Vitamin A metabolism: an update. 2011 Nutrients;3(1):63-103.

De Andrade JAA, Gayer CRM, Nogueira NPA, Paes MC et al. The effect of thiamine deficiency and inflammation, oxidative stress and cellular migration in an experimental model of sepsis. 2014 J Inflamm;11.11

De Farias CR, Cardoso BR, de Oliveira GM, de Mello Guazzelli IC, et al. A randomized-controlled, double-blind study of the impact of selenium supplementation on thyroid autoimmunity and inflammation with focus on the GPx1 genotypes. 2015 J Endocrinol Invest;38(1):1065-74.

Eftekhari M, Keshavarz S. Jalali M. Elguero E. et.al. The relationship between iron status and thyroid hormone concentration in iron-deficient adolescent Iranian girls. 2006 Asia Pac J Clin Nutr;15(1):50-5.

Ergas D, Eilat E, Mendlovic S, Sthoeger ZM. N-3 fatty acids and the immune system in autoimmunity. 2002 Isr Med Assoc J;4(1):34-8.

Farhangi MA, Dehghan P, Tajmiri S, Abbasi MM. The effects of Nigella sativa on thyroid function, serum Vascular Endothelial Growth Factor (VEGF) - 1, Nesfatin-1 and anthropometric features in patients with Hashimoto's thyroiditis: a randomized controlled trial. 2016 BMC Complement Altern Med;16(1):471.

Farhangi MA, Keshavarz SA, Eshraghian M, Ostadrahimi A, Saboor-Yaraghi AA. The effect of vitamin a supplementation every function in premenopausal women. 2012 J Am Coll Nutr;31(4):268-74.

Flagg EW, Coates RJ, Eley JW, Jones DP, Gunter EW, Byers TE, Block GS, Greenberg RS. Dietary glutathione intake in humans and the relationship between intake and plasma total glutathione level. 1994 Nutr Cancer;21(1):33-46.

Gartner R, Gasnier BC, Dietrich JW, Krebs B, et al. Selenium supplementation in patients with autoimmune thyroiditis decreases thyroid peroxidase antibody concentrations. 2002 J Clin Endocrinol Metab;87(4):1687-1691.

Ghorbanibirgani A, Khalili A, Rokhafrooz D. Comparing Nigella sativa Oil and fish oil in treatment of vitiligo. 2014 Iran Red Crescent Med J;16(6):e4515.

Giuliani C, Iezzi M, Ciolli L, Hysi A, et al. Resveratrol has anti-thyroid effects both in vitro and in vivo. 2017 Food Chem Toxicol;107(Pt A):37-247.

Guo Y, Wan SY, Zhong X, Zhong MK, Pan TR. Levothyroxine replacement therapy with vitamin D supplementation prevents the oxidative stress and apoptosis in hippocampus of hypothyroid rats. 2014 Neuro Endocrinol Lett;35(8):684-90.

Hadi V, Kheirouri S, Alizadeh M, Khabbazi A, Hosseini H. effects of Nigella sativa oil extract on a inflammatory cytokine response and oxidative stress status in patients with rheumatoid arthritis: a randomized, double-blind, placebo-controlled clinical trial. 2016 Avicenna J Phytomed;6(1):34-43.

Jafarpour SM, Safaei M, Mohseni M, Salimian M, et al. The Radioprotective Effects of Curcumin and Trehalose Against Genetic Damage Caused By I-131. 2018 Indian J Nucl Me.;33(2):99-104.

Johannes J, Jayarama-Naidu R, Meyer F, Wirth EK, et al. Silychristin, a Flavonolignan Derived From the Milk Thistle, Is a Potent Inhibitor of the Thyroid Hormone Transporter MCT8. 2016 Endocrinology;157(4):1694-701.

Kasahara H, Kondo T, Nakatsukasa H, Chikuma S, Ito M, Ando M, Kurebayashi Y, Sekiya T, Yamada T, Okamoto S, Yoshimura A. Generation of allo-antigen-specific induced Treg stabilized by vitamin C treatment and its application for prevention of acute graft versus host disease model. 2017 Int Immunol;29(10):457-469.

Kiseleva EP1, Mikhailopulo KI, Sviridov OV, Novik GI, Knirel YA, Szwajcer Dey E. The role of components of Bifidobacterium and Lactobacillus in pathogenesis and serologic diagnosis of autoimmune thyroiddiseases. 2011 Benef Microbes;2(2):139-54.

Latrofa F, Fiore E, Rago T, Antonangeli L, et al. Iodine contributes to thyroid autoimmunity in humans by unmasking a cryptic epitope on thyroglobulin. 2013 J Clin Endocrinol Metab;98(11):E1768-74.

Liu H, Zheng T, Mao Y, Xu C, Bu L, Mou X, Zhou Y, Yuan G, Wang S, Zhou T, Chen D, Mao C. γδ T cells enhance B cells for antibody production and Hashimoto's thyroiditis, and retinoic acid induces apoptosis of the γδ T cell. Endocrine. 2016 Jan;51(1):113-22.

Lukienko Pl, Mel'nichenko NG, Zverinskii IV, Zabrodskaya SV. Antioxidant properties of thiamine. 2000 Bull Exp Biol Med;130(9):874-6.

Majdalawieh AF, Fayyad MW. Immunomodulary and anti-inflammatory action of Nigella sativa and thymoquinone: A comprehensive review. 2015 Int Immunopharmacol;28(1):295-304.

Mazokopakis EE, Papadomanolaki MG, Tsekouras KC, Evangelopoulous AD, Kotsiris DA, Tzortzinis AA. Is vitamin D related to pathogenesis and treatment of Hashimoto's thyroiditis? 2015 Hell J Nucl Med;18(3):222-7.

McCarty MF. Upregulation of lymphocyte apoptosis as a strategy for preventing and treating autoimmune disorders: a rule for whole-food vegan diets, fish oil and dopamine agonists. 2001 Med Hypotheses;57(2):358-75.

Mennen LI, Walker R, Bennetau-Pelissero C, Scalbert A. Risks and safety of polyphenol consumption. 2005 Am J Clin Nutr;81(1 Suppl):26S-329S.

Nourbakhsh M, Ahmadpour F, Chahardoli B, Malekpour-Dehkordi Z, et al. Selenium and its relationship with selenoprotein P and glutathione peroxidase in children and adolescents with Hashimoto's thyroiditis and hypothyroidism. 2016 J Trace Elem Med Biol;34:10-14.

Office of Dietary Supplements - Zinc [Internet]. NIH Office of Dietary Supplements. U.S. Department of Health and Human Services; 2016 [Cited 17 Aug 2018]. Available from: https://ods.od.nih.gov/factsheets/Zinc-Consumer/

Ogungbe IV, Crouch RA, Demeritte T. (-) Arctigenin and (+) Pinoresinol Are Antagonists of the Human Thyroid Hormone Receptor B. 2014 J Chem Inf Model; 54(11):3051-55.

Panda S, Kar A. Changes in thyroid hormone concentrations after administration of ashwagandharoot extract to adult male mice. 1998 J Pharm Pharmacol;50(9):1065-8.

Panda S, Kar A. Evidence for free radical scavenging activity of Ashwagandha root powder in mice. 1997 Indian J Physiol Pharmacol;41(4):424-6.

Premawardhana LD, Parkes AB, Smyth PP, Wijeyaratne CN et al. Increased prevalence of thyroglobulin antibodies in Sri Lankan schoolgirls—is iodine the cause? 2000 Eur J Endocrinol;143(2):185-8.

Prietl B, Treiber G, Pieber TR, Amrein K.

Vitamin D and immune function. 2013 Nutritents;5(7):2502-21.

Richie JP Jr, Nichenametla S, Neidig W, Calcagnotto A, et al. Randomized controlled trial of oral glutathione supplementation on body stores of glutathione. 2015 Eur J Nutr;54(2):251-63.

Rosario PW, Batista KC, Calsolari MR. Radio iodine-induced oxidative stress in patients with different to their carcinoma and effective supplementation with vitamin C and E and selenium (antioxidants). 2016 Arch Endocrinol Metab;60(4):328-32.

Schwertheim S, Wein F, Lennartz K, Worm K, et al. Curcumin induces G2/M arrest, apoptosis, NF- B inhibition, and expression of differentiation genes in thyroid carcinoma cells. 2017 J Cancer Res Clin Oncol;143(7):1143-1154.

Segermann J, Hotze A, Ulrich H, Rao GS. Effect of alpha-lipoic acid on the peripheral conversion of thyroxine to triiodothyronine and on serum lipid-, protein- and glucose levels. 1991 Arzneimittelforschung;41(12):1294-8.

Shan Z, Chen L, Lian X, Liu C, et al. Iodine Status and Prevalence of Thyroid disorders after introduction of mandatory universal salt Iodization for 16 years in China: a cross-sectional study in 10 Cities. 2016 Thyroid;26(8):1125-30.

Sharma AK, Basu I, Singh S. Efficacy and Safety of Ashwagandha Root Extract in Subclinical Hypothyroid Patients: A Double-Blind, Randomized Placebo-Controlled Trial. 2018 J Altern Complement Med;24(3):243-248.

Simopoulos AP. Omega-3 fatty acids in inflammation and autoimmune diseases. 2002 J Am Coll Nutr; 21(6):495-505.

Soliman AT1, De Sanctis V, Yassin M, Wagdy M, Soliman N. Chronic anemia and thyroid function. 2017 Acta Biomed;88(1):119-127.

Spinas E, Saggini A, Kritas Sk, Cerulli G,

Caraffa A, Antinolfi P ,Pantalone A, Frydas A, Tei M, Speziali A, Saggini R, Pandolfi F, Conti P. Can vitamin A mediate immunity and inflammation? 2015 J Biol Regul Homeost Agents;29(1):1-6.

Stephensen CB. Vitamin A, infection, and immune function. 2001 Annu Rev Nutr;21: 167-92.

Taddei S, Caraccio N, Virdis A, Dardano A, Versari D, Ghiadoni L, Ferrannini E, Salvetii A, Monzani F. Low-grade systemic inflammation causes endothelial dysfunctiom in patients with Hashimoto's thyroiditis. 2006 J Clin Endocrinol Metab;91(12):5076-82.

Tan L, Sang Z, Shen J, Liu H, et al. Prevalence of thyroid dysfunction with adequate and excessive iodine intake in Hebei Province, People's Republic of China. 2015 Public Health Nutr;18(9):1692-7.

Toulis KA, Anastasilakis AD, Tzellos TG, Goulis DG, Kouvelas D. selenium supplementation in the treatment of Hashimoto's thyroiditis: a systematic review and a meta-analysis. 2010 Thyroid;20(10):1163-73.

Trochoutsou Al, Kloukina V, Samitas K, Xanthou G. Vitamin-D in the Immune System: Genomic and Non-Genomic Actions. 2015 Mini Rev Med CheM;15(11):953-63.

Venditti P, Di Stefano L, Di Meo S. vitamin E management of oxidative damage linked dysfunctions of hyperthyroid tissue. 2013 Cell Mol Life Sci;70(17):3125-44.

Vlasova AN, Kandasamy S, Chattha KS, Rajashekara G et al. Comparison of probiotic lactobacilli and bifidobacteria effects, immune responses and rotavirus vaccines and infection in different host species. 2018 Vet Immunol Immunopathol;172:72-84.

Vondra K, Starka L, Hampl R. Vitamin D and thyroid diseases. 2015 Physiol Res;64(2):S95-S100.

Witschi A, Reddy S, Stofer B, Lauterburg BH. The systemic availability of oral glutathione. 1992 Eur J Clin Pharmacol;43(6):667-9.

Yang P, Li Y, Xu G. Antioxidant therapy improves non-thyroidal illness syndrome in uremic rats. 2016 Ren Fail;38(4):514-20.

Yu J, Shan Z, Chong W, Mao J, Geng Y, Zhang C, Xing Q, Wang W, Li N, Fan C, Wang H, Zhang H, Teng W. Vitamin E ameliorates iodine-induced cytotoxicity and thyroid. 2011 J Endocrinol;209(3):299-306.

Zimmerman MB, Kohrle J. The impact of iron in selenium deficiencies and iodine and thyroid metabolism: biochemistry and relevance to public health. 2002 Thyroid;12(10):867-78.

Chapter 11

Agate L et al. Thyroid Autoantibodies and Thyroid Function in Subjects Exposed to Chernobyl Fallout during Childhood: Evidence for a Transient Radiation-Induced Elevation of Serum Thyroid Antibodies without an Increase in Thyroid Autoimmune Disease. 2008 The Journal of Clinical Endocrinology & Metabolism;93(7):2729-2736.

Aker AM, Watkins DJ, Johns LE, Ferguson KK, Soldin OP, Anzalota Del Toro LV, Alshawabkeh AN, Cordero JF, Meeker JD. Phenols and parabens in relation to reproductive and thyroid hormones in pregnant women. 2016 Environ Res;151:30-37.

Bassi V, Marino G, Iengo A, Fattoruso O, Santinelli C. Autoimmune thyroid diseases and Helicobacter pylori: the correlation is present only in Graves's disease. 2012 World J Gastroenterol;18(10):1093-7.

Becker NP, Braun D, Hoefig CS, Köhrle J, Renko K, Schäche S, Schomburg L, Schweibert C, Welsnik T. An Improved Nonradioactive Screening Method Identifies Genistein and Xanthohumol as Potent Inhibitors of Iodothyronine Deiodinases. 2015 Thyroid;25(8):962-8.

Benvenga S et al. Type of fish consumed and thyroid autoimmunity in pregnancy and postpartum. 2016 Endocrine;52:120-129.

Bernatsky S, Smargiassi A, Joseph L et al. Industrial air emissions, and proximity to major industrial emitters, are associated with anti-citrullinated protein antibodies. 2017 Environ Res;157:60-63.

Bigazzi PE. Metals and Kidney Autoimmunity. 1999 Environ Health Perspect;107 Suppl 5:753-65.

Blount BC, Pirkle JL, Osterloh JD, Valentin-Blasini L, Caldwell K. Urinary perchlorate in thyroid hormone levels in adolescent and adult men and women living in the United States. 2006 Environ Health Perspect;114:1865-1871.

Chailurkit La-or, Aekplakorn W e tal. The Association of Serum Bisphenol A with Thyroid Autoimmunity. 2016 B Int J Environ Res Public Health;13(11):1153.

Chen A, Kim S, Chung E, Dietrich K. Thyroid Hormones in Relation to Lead, Mercury, and Cadmium Exposure in the National Health and Nutrition Examination Survey, 2007-2008. 2013 Environ Health Perspect;121.

Chevrier J. Gunier RB, Bradman A, Holland NT, Calafat AM, Eskenazi B, Harley KG. Maternal urinary bisphenol a during pregnancy and maternal and neonatal thyroid function in the CHAMACOS study. 2013 Environ Health PerspecT;121(1):138-44.

Cho YA, Kim J. Thyroid cancer risk and smoking status: a meta-analysis. 2014 CCC;25(9):1187-95.

Claus SP, Guillou H, Ellero-Simatos S. The gut microbiota: a major player in the toxicity of environment pollutants? 2017 Biofilms Microbiomes;3:17001.

Costenbader KH. 2006 Lupus;15(11):737-745.

Cui H1, Xu B, Wu T, Xu J, Yuan Y, Gu Q. Potential antiviral lignans from the roots of Saururus chinensis with activity against Epstein-Barr virus lytic replication. 2014 J Nat Prod;77(1):100-10.

Cutolo M et al. Estrogen metabolism and autoimmunity. 2012 Autoimmunity Reviews;11(6-7):A460-464.

DiGangi J, Blum A, Bergman Å, et al. San

Antonio Statement on Brominated and Chlorinated Flame Retardants. 2010 Environmental Health Perspectives;118(12):A516-A518.

Tribune Watchdog: Playing With Fire [Internet]. Chicago Tribune [Cited 17 Aug 2018]. Available from: http://media.apps.chicagotribune.com/flames/index.html

Dufault R, Schnoll R, Lukiw W, LeBlanc B, Cornett C, Patrick L, Wallinga D, Gilbert S, Crider R. Mercury exposure, nutritional deficiencies and metabolic disruptions may affect learning in children. 2009 Behav Brain Funct;5:44.

Environmental Protection Agency. Basic Information on PFAS [Internet]. EPA; 2018 [Cited 17 Aug 2018]. Available from: https://www.epa.gov/pfas/basic-information-pfas

Farhat SC et al. Air pollution in autoimmune rheumatic diseases: a review. 2011 Autoimmun Rev;11(1):14-21

Fuggle NR, Smith TO, Kual A, Sofat N. Hand to Mouth: a Systematic Review and Meta-analysis of the Association Between Rheumatoid Arthritis and Periodontitis. 2016 Front Immunol;7(80).

Gallagher CM, Meliker JR. Mercury and thyroid autoantibodies in U.S. women, NHANES 2007-2008. 2012 Environ Int.;40:39-43.

Guo Q, Sun X, Zhang Z, Zhang L, Yao G, Li F, Yang X, Song L, Jiang G. The effect of Astragalus polysaccharide on the Epstein-Barr virus lytic cycle. 2014 Acta Virol;58(1):76-80.

Henley DV, Lipson N, Korach KS, Bloch CA. Prepubertal gynecomastia linked to lavender and tea tree oils. 2007 N Engl J Med;356(5):479-85.

Imhann F et al. Proton pump inhibitors affect the gut microbiome. 2016 Gut;65:740-748.

Jancic SA. Cadmium and thyroid. 2014 Vitam Horm;94:391-42.

Kapu ci ska A, Nowak I. The use of phytoestrogens in anti-ageing cosmetics. 2015 Chemik;3:154-159.

Khan MF, Wang G. Environmental Agents, Oxidative Stress and Autoimmunity. 2018 Curr Opin Toxicol;7:22-27

Kim J, Bang Y, Lee WJ. Living near nuclear power plants and thyroid cancer risk: A systematic review and meta-analysis. 2016 Environment international;87:42-48.

Kisakol G. Dental amalgam implantation and thyroid autoimmunity. 2014 Bratisl Lek Listy;115(1):22-4.

Koeppe ES, Ferguson KK, Colacino JA, Meeker JD. Relationship between urinary triclosan and paraben concentrations and serum thyroid measures in NHANES 2007-2008. 2013 Sci Total Environ;445-446:299-305.

Kurien BT, Hensley K, Bachmann M, Scofield RH. Autoimmunity and oxidatively modified autoantigens. 2006 Free Rad Biol Med;41:549-556.

Leonidas H, Duntas and Nikos Stathatos. Toxic chemicals and thyroid function: hard facts and lateral thinking. 2015 Rev Endocr Metab Disord;16:311-318.

Mikuls TR, et al. Periodontitis and Porphyromonas gingivalis in Patients with Rheumatoid Arthritis. Arthritis Rheumatol. 2014 May;66(5):1090-1100.

Mohammad I, Starskaia I, Nagy T, Guo J, Yatkin E, Väänänen K, Watford WT, Chen Z/. Estrogen receptor Alpha contributes to T cell mediated auto immune inflammation by promoting T-cell activation and proliferation. 2018 Sci Signal;11(526).

Patisaul HB, Jefferson W. The Pros and Cons of Phytoestrogens. 2010 Front Neuroendocrinol;31(4):400-419.

Patrick L. Thyroid disruption: mechanism and clinical implications in human health. 2009 Altern Med Rev;14(4):326-46.

Pellegriti G, et al. Papillary thyroid cancer

incidence in the volcanic area of Sicily. 2009 J Natl Cancer Inst;101(22):1575-83.

Malandrino P, Russo M, Ronchi A, Minoia C, Cataldo D, Regalbuto C, Giordano C, Attard M, Squatrito S, Trimarchi F, Vigneri R. Increased thyroid cancer incidence in a basaltic volcanic area is associated with non-anthropogenic pollution and biocontamination. 2016 Endocrine;53(2):471-9.

Pinkerton LE, Hein MJ, Anderson JL, Christianson A, Little MP, Sigurdson AJ, Schubauer-Berigan MK. Melanoma, thyroid cancer, and gynecologic cancers in a cohort of female flight attendants. 2018 Am J Ind Med;61(7):572-581.

Pfau JC et al. Nested Case-Control Study of Autoimmune Disease in an Asbestos-Exposed Population. 2005 Environ Health Perspect;113:25-30

Pfau JC, Serve KM, Noonan CW. Autoimmunity and asbestos exposure. 2014 Autoimmune Dis;2014:782045.

Russo M, Malandrino P, Addario WP, Dardanoni G, Vigneri P, Pellegriti G, Squatrito S, Vigneri R. Several Site-specific Cancers are Increased in the Volcanic Area in Sicily. 2015 Anticancer Res;35(7):3995-4001.

Sawicka-Gutaj N, Gutaj P, Sowi ski J, Wender-O egowska E, Czarnywojtek A, Br zert J, Ruchała M. Influence of cigarette smoking on thyroid gland--an update. 2014 Endokrynol Pol;65(1):54-62.

Shi WJ, Liu W, Zhou XY, Ye F, Zhang GX. Associations of Helicobacter pylori infection and cytotoxin-associated gene A status with autoimmune thyroid diseases: a meta-analysis. 2013 Thyroid;23(10):1294-300.

Shukla SK, Singh G, Ahmad S, Pant P. Infections, genetic and environmental factors in pathogenesis of autoimmune thyroid diseases. 2018 Microb Pathog;116:279-288.

Montenegro L, et al. Nonsteroidal Anti-Inflammatory Drug Induced Damage on Lower Gastro-Intestinal Tract: Is There an Involvement of Microbiota? 2014 Curr Drug Saf;9(3):196-204.

Wojciech Marlicz et al. Nonsteroidal Anti-Inflammatory Drugs, Proton Pump Inhibitors, and Gastrointestinal Injury: Contrasting Interactions in the Stomach and Small Intestine. 2014 Mayo Clin Proc;89(12):1699-1709.

Sigaux J, et al. Air pollution as a determinant of rheumatoid arthritis. 2018 Joint Bone Spine;S1297-319X(18)30043-5.

The Use of Cadmium and Its Compounds in Articles Coloured for Safety Reasons [Internet]. European Chemicals Agency (ECHA); 9 Nov 2012. Available from: https://echa. europa.eu/documents/10162/13641/ cadmium_articles_coloured_safety_reasons_201201_en.pdf/8bfae53a-d988-4568-b3bd-992790a718c9

Toussirot E, Roudier J. Epstein-Barr virus in autoimmune diseases. Best Practice & Research. 2008 Clin Rheum;22(5):883-96.

Tsuda T, Tokinobu A, Yamamoto E, Suzuki E. nThyroid cancer detection by ultrasound among residents ages 18 years and younger in Fukushima, Japan: 2011 to 2014. 2016 Epidemiology 27(3):316.

Valesini G, Schoenfeld Y, et al. Citrullination and autoimmunity. 2015 Autoimmun Rev;14(6):490-7

Wang S, Wang Y. Peptidylarginine deiminases in citrullination, gene regulation, health and pathogenesis. 2013 Biochim Biophys Acta;1829(10):1126-35.

Webber M, Moir W, Crowson C, Cohen H, Zeig-Owens R, Hall C, Berman J, Qayyum B, Jaber N, RPA-C, Matteson E, Liu Y, Kelly K, Prezant D. Post-September 11, 2001, Incidence of Systemic Autoimmune Diseases in World Trade Center—Exposed Firefighters and Emergency Medical Service Workers. 2016 Mayo Clin Proc;91(1):23-32.

Zihlif MA, Mahmoud IS, Ghanim MT, Zreikat MS, Alrabadi N, Imraish A, Odeh F, Abbas MA, Ismail SI. Thymoquinone efficiently inhibits the survival of EBV-infected B cells and alters EBV gene expression. 2013 Integr Cancer Ther;12(3):257-63.

Chapter 12

Atanackovic D, Nowottne U, Freier E, Weber CS, Meyer S, Bartels K, Hildebrandt Y, Cao Y, Kröger N, Brunner-Weinzierl MC, Bokemeyer C, Deter HC. Acute psychological stress increases peripheral blood CD3+CD56+ natural killer T cells in healthy men: possible implications for the development and treatment of allergic and autoimmune disorders. 2013 Stress;16(4):421-8.

Birdsall, T. C. 5-Hydroxytryptophan: A Clinically-Effective Serotonin Precursor. 1998 Altern Med Rev;3(4):271-280.

Bolk N, Visser TJ, Nijman J. Effects of Evening vs Morning Levothyroxine Intake: A Randomized Double-blind Crossover Trial. 2010 Arch Intern Med;170(22):1996-2003.

Sorells SF, Sapolsky RM. An Inflammatory Review of Glucocorticoid Actions in the CNS. 2007 Brain Behav Immunr;21(3):259-72.

Damian L, Ghiciuc CM, Dima-Cozma LC, et al. No definitive evidence for a connection between autoimmune thyroid diseases and stress in women. 2017 Activitas Nervosa Superior Rediviva;59(1).

Dhabhar FS, Viswanathan K. Short-term stress experienced at time of immunization induces a long-lasting increase in immunologic memory. 2005 Am J Physiol Regul Integr Comp Physiol; 289(3):R738-44.

Dhabhar FS. Enhancing versus suppressive effects of stress on immune function: implications for immunoprotection and immunopathology. 2009 Neuroimmunomodulation;16(5):300-17.

Effraimidis G, Tijssen JG, Brosschot JF, Wiersinga WM. Involvement of stress in the pathogenesis of autoimmune thyroid disease: a prospective study. 2010 Psychoneuroendocrinology;37(8):1191-8.

Fux M, Levine BJ, Aviv A, Belmaker RH.

Inositol Treatment Of Obsessive-Compulsive Disorder. 1996 Am J Psychiatry;153(9):1219.

Krysiak R, Kowalcze K, Okopien B. The effect of statin therapy on thyroid autoimmunity in patients with Hashimoto's thyroiditis: A pilot study. 2016 Pharmacol Rep;68(2):429-33.

Krysiak R, Szkrobka W, Okopien B. The Effect of Vitamin D on Thyroid Autoimmunity in Levothyroxine-Treated Women with Hashimoto's Thyroiditis and Normal Vitamin D Status. 2017 Exp Clin Endocrinol Diabetes;125(4):229-233.

Kulkarni SK. Heat and other physiological stress-induced analgesia: catecholamine mediated and naloxone reversible response. Life Sci. 1980 Jul 21;27(3):185-8.

Liwanpo L, Hershman JM. Conditions and drugs interfering with thyroxine absorption. Best Pract Res Clin Endocrinol Metab. 2009 Dec; 23(6):781-92.

Lynch T, Price A. The Effect of Cytochrome P450 Metabolism on Drug Response, Interactions and Adverse Effects. 2007 Am Fam Physician;76(3):391-396.

Microbiology by numbers [Internet]. Editorial. 2011 Nature;9.

Moroda T, Kawachi Y, Iiai T, Tsukahara A, Suzuki S, Tada T, Watanabe H, Hatakeyama K, Abo T Self-reactive forbidden clones are confined to pathways of intermediate T-cell receptor cell differentiation even under immunosuppressive conditions. 1997 Immunology; 91(1):88-94.

Nobuyuki T, Yamada T, Takasu M, Komiya I, Nagasawa Y, Asawa T, Shinoda T, Aizawa T, Koizumi Y. Disappearance of Thyrotropin-Blocking Antibodies and Spontaneous Recovery from Hypothyroidism in Autoimmune Thyroiditis. 1992 N Engl J Med;326:513-518

Prietl B, et al. High-dose cholecalciferol supplementation significantly increases peripheral CD4 Tregs in healthy adults without negatively affecting the frequency of other immune cells. 2013 Eur J Nutr;53(3):761-9

Rao R, Samak G. Role of Glutamine in Protection of Intestinal Epithelial Tight Junctions. 2012 J Epithel Biol Pharmacol;5(Suppl 1-M7):47-54.

Sawicka-Gutaj N, Gutaj P, Sowinski J, Wender-Ozegowska E, et al. Influence of cigarette smoking on thyroid gland—an update. 2014 Endokrynol Pol;65(1):52-62.

Shri, R. Anxiety: Causes and Management. 2010 IBJS;5(1).

Sorrells SF, Sapolsky RM. An inflammatory review of glucocorticoid actions in the CNS. Stress. 2013 Jul;16(4):421-8.

Van Zuuren EJ, Albusta AY, Fedorowicz Z, Carter B, Pijl H. Selenium supplementation for Hashimoto's thyroiditis. 2013 Cochrane Database Syst Rev;(6):CD010223.

Velickovic D, Veljkovic M. The Study of Vitamins B1,B6, and B12 Effects on Adrenal Cortex Adaptation By Monitoring Some Enzyme System Rats Trained by Swimming. 2014 Medfak;UDC:612.45-015.1:577.164.1.

Veru F, Laplante DP, Luheshi G, King S. Prenatal maternal stress exposure and immune function in the offspring. 2014 Stress;17(2):133-48.

Xu C, Wu F, Mao C, Wang X, et al. Excess iodine promotes apoptosis of thyroid follicular epithelial cells by inducing autophagy suppression and is associated with Hashimoto thyroiditis disease. 2016 J Autoimmun;75:50-57.

Chapter 13

Adam MA, Thomas S, Youngwirth L, Hyslop T, Reed SD, Scheri RP, Roman SA, Sosa JA. Is There a Minimum Number of Thyroidectomies a Surgeon Should Perform to Optimize Patient Outcomes? 2017 Ann Surg;265(2):402-407.

Bagley D. January 2016: Thyroid Month: The Saga of Radioactive Therapy [Internet]. Endocrine News; Jan 2016. Available from: https://endocrinenews.endocrine.org/january-2016-thyroid-month-the-saga-of-radioiodine-therapy/

Hamidi O, Callstrom MR, Lee RA, Dean D, Castro R, Morris JC, Stan MN. Outcomes of Radiofrequency Ablation Therapy for Large Benign Thyroid Nodules: A Mayo Clinic Case Series. 2018 Mayo Clin Proc;93(8):1018-1025.

Kovatcheva RD, Vlahov JD, Stoinov JI, Zaletel K. Benign Solid Thyroid Nodules: US-guided High-Intensity Focused Ultrasound Ablation-Initial Clinical Outcomes. 2015 Radiology;276(2):597-605.

Resources

THYROID AND AUTOIMMUNE RELATED ORGANIZATIONS

General Hashimoto's Information

Additional information on Hashimoto's disease can be found at the following websites and foundations:

American Thyroid Association (ATA)

6066 Leesburg Pike #550
Falls Church, VA 22041
ATA has over 1,700 members comprised of physicians and scientists, and is dedicated to the many aspects of thyroid disorders and cancer.
Website: www.thyroid.org/hashimotos-thyroiditis
Email: thyroid@thyroid.org
Phone: 703-998-8890

National Institutes of Health (NIH)

Clinical Center
10 Center Drive
Bethesda, MD 20814
The NIH is the largest biomedical research agency in the world, and is an agency of the U.S. Department of Health and Human Services.
Website: www.niddk.nih.gov/health-information/endocrine-diseases/hashimotos-disease
Phone: 800-860-8747

Thyroid Cancer

Thyroid cancer patients can find additional information and support at the following websites:

Thyroid Cancer Survivors' Association (ThyCa)

Created and maintained by patients, ThyCa links thyroid cancer patients/survivors and health care professionals worldwide. ThyCa offers an array of resources and information for people with thyroid cancer and their loved ones. The organization also provides its members with an online forum for the exchange of information and support.
Website: www.thyca.org
Email: thyca@thyca.org
Phone: 877-588-7904

ThyCa Low Iodine Diet Information

The following link will direct you to ThyCa's extensive set of guidelines and information, including a cookbook (see below), for people preparing to receive radioactive iodine (RAI) for thyroid cancer tests.
Website: www.thyca.org/pap-fol/lowiodinediet/

ThyCa Low Iodine Diet Cookbook

ThyCa's free Low Iodine Diet Cookbook contains over four hundred low-iodine recipes and diet guidelines from medical professionals. Print the cookbook or download the PDF to your computer, phone, or tablet at the following link: www.thyca.org/download/document/231/Cookbook.pdf

Thyroid Cancer Connect

Thyroid Cancer Connect is an online support group where you can engage in discussions on a wide variety of topics relating to thyroid cancer with other members of the ThyCa community.

Website: www.inspire.com/groups/thyca-thyroid-cancer-survivors-association

Email: team@inspire.com

Phone: 800-945-0381

National Cancer Institute (NCI)

9609 Medical Center Drive

Rockville, MD 20850

NCI is part of the NIH and is dedicated to research, training, and other programs related to the cause, diagnosis, prevention, and treatment of cancer.

General Website: www.cancer.gov

Website (Thyroid Cancer): www.cancer.gov/types/thyroid

Website (Clinical Trials): www.cancer.gov/about-cancer/treatmnet/clinical-trials/search

Phone: 800-422-6237

Thyroid Diagnostic Procedures

These websites provide information for patients related to thyroid diagnostic procedures.

MedlinePlus

MedlinePlus is the NIH's website, containing the world's largest medical library.

Thyroid Ultrasound

Website: https://medlineplus.gov/ency/article/003776.htm

Radiologyinfo.org

Radiologyinfo.org is a resource that has information regarding radiological procedures, including preparation and what patients can expect. The website includes diagnostic and interventional radiology, nuclear medicine, and radiation therapy.

Thyroid Uptake & Scan

Website: www.radiologyinfo.org/en/info.cfm?PG=thyroiduptake

Fine Needle Thyroid Biopsy

Website: www.radiologyinfo.org/en/info.cfm?pg=thyroidbiopsy

Thyroid Organizations

There are specific thyroid organizations dedicated to the advancement of thyroid education, research and knowledge.

Graves' Disease & Thyroid Foundation

P.O. Box 2793

Rancho Santa Fe, CA 92067

The Graves' & Thyroid Foundation educates and supports patients, caregivers, and healthcare professionals.

Website: www.gdatf.org

Email: info@gdatf.org

Phone: 877-643-3123

National Academy of Hypothyroidism

The National Academy of Hypo-thyroidism is made up of a group of thyroidologists dedicated to disseminating information about the diagnosis and treatment of treatment of hypothyroidism.

Website: www.nahypothyroidism.org

Email (Contact Form): https://www.nahypothyroidism.org/contact-us

Thyroid Change

An international advocacy website, encompassing a community of medical professionals and patients concerned with thyroid patient care.

Website: http://www.thyroidchange.org

Find a Doctor: http://www.thyroidchange.org/find-a-doctor1.html

Email: thyroidchange@gmail.com

For Non-Thyroid Autoimmune Illnesses

People with autoimmune thyroid disease may have other associated autoimmune conditions. The following organizations provide infomation and support for patients who are suffering with various forms of autoimmunity. All of the following groups are dedicated to helping patients by offering a variety of services and information.

Arthritis

Rheumatoid Arthritis

American College of Rheumatology

2200 Lake Boulevard NE
Atlanta, GA 30319

The American College of Rheumatology is an organization of over 9,400 rheumatologists and other health professionals involved in the education, treatment, and research of hematological diseases and conditions.

Website: www.rheumatology.org/I-Am-A/Patient-Caregiver/Diseases-Conditions/Rheumatoid-Arthritis

Phone: 404-633-3777

The Arthritis Foundation

1355 Peachtree St NE
Suite 600
Atlanta, GA 30309

The Arthritis Foundation is a comprehensive organization that improves the lives of arthritis patients through information and resources.

Website: www.arthritis.org/about-arthritis/types/rheumatoid-arthritis/what-is-rheumatoid-arthritis.php

Phone (Helpline): 844-571-4357

Lupus

The Lupus Foundation of America

2121 K Street NW, Suite 200
Washington, DC 20037

The Lupus Foundation of America provides caring support for those with lupus, as they try to solve the mystery of the disease. They have several chapters/groups throughout the country.

Website: www.lupus.org

Find a Chapter: https://www.lupus.org/chapters

Email: info@lupus.org

Phone: 800-558-0121

Lupus Research Alliance

275 Madison Avenue, 10th Floor
New York, NY 10016

The Lupus Research Alliance describes themselves as the "world's leading private funder of lupus research." The website has sections on research and clinical trials, a lupus community, and resources, among others.

Website: www.lupusresearch.org
Phone: 800-867-1743

Autoimmune Diseases

American Autoimmune Related Diseases Association (AARDA)
22100 Gratiot Avenue
Eastpointe, MI 48021
AARDA describes itself as the "only national nonprofit" focused on helping those who affected by over 100 different autoimmune related conditions.

Website: www.aarda.org
Email: aarda@aarda.org
Phone: 800-598-4668

Celiac Disease

Celiac Disease Foundation
20350 Ventura Boulevard, Suite 240
Woodland Hills, CA 91364
The Celiac Disease Foundation is focused on accelerating the diagnosis, treatment and cure for those with celiac disease and wheat sensitivity.

Website: https://celiac.org
Website (Contact Form): celiac.org/contact-us
Phone: 818-716-1513

Chronic Fatigue Syndrome

The Solve ME/CFS Initiative (SMCI)
5455 Wilshire Blvd, Ste 1903
Los Angeles, CA 90036-0007
Website: https://solvecfs.org

Email: SolveCFS@SolveCFS.org
Phone: 704-364-0016

Diabetes

American Diabetes Association
2451 Crystal Drive, Suite 900
Arlington, VA 22202
The American Diabetes Association funds research, delivers services, provides information, and advocates for those dealing with diabetes.

Website: www.diabetes.org/diabetes-basics/type-1
Email: askADA@diabetes.org
Phone: 800.DIABETES (800-342-2383)

Fibromyalgia

National Fibromyalgia & Chronic Pain Association (NFMCPA)
31 Federal Avenue
Logan, UT 84321
NFMCPA unites communities of patients, policy makers, and those in the medical/scientific fields to work toward ending chronic pain conditions (including fibromyalgia).

Website: www.fmaware.org
Email: info@fmcpaware.org
Phone: 801-200-3627

Multiple Sclerosis

National MS Society
The National MS Society mobilizes people and resources to help those affected by multiple sclerosis.

Website: www.nationalmssociety.org
Find a Location Near You: https://www.nationalmssociety.org/Chapters
Phone: 800-344-4867

AITD Online Support

Online communities are a valuable resource for Hashimoto's patients, as well as those will other thyroid issues. Always remember that while these websites can be extremely helpful for gaining information, support, and the exchange of ideas, they are not meant to take the place of getting help from your own provider.

ChronicBabe

A popular multi-platform resource created by a woman with multiple chronic disorders for women for chronic health conditions, including thyroid issues.
Website: www.chronicbabe.com

Doctor Thyroid with Philip James

Although the host of this podcast is not a doctor, he interviews many doctors in the field of thyroid disease, including endocrinologists, surgeons, and pathologists.
Website: https://docthyroid.com

Hypothyroid Mom

One woman's experience with hypothyroidism evolved into an enormously popular website/blog and Facebook page—with over 1 million followers. She has and continues to raise awareness about the complex world of hypothyroidism.
Website: https://hypothyroidmom.com
Facebook page: www.facebook.com/HypothyroidMom

Inspire.com

3101 Wilson Boulevard, Suite 220
Arlington, VA 22201
Inspire.com is a social network where patients can connect with each other for support and information. Along with forums on various thyroid conditions, they also have forums on several other autoimmune diseases.
Email: team@inspire.com
Phone: 800-945-0381

Thyroid Disease Forum: https://www.inspire.com/groups/thyroid-diseases

Thyroid Cancer Forum: https://www.inspire.com/groups/thyca-thyroid-cancer-survivors-association

Thyroid Boards—Hashimoto's Message Board

Thyroidboards.com is a collection of different message forums related to a variety of thyroid topics.
Website: http://thyroidboards.com/forums/forum/5-hashimotos-thyroiditis-hashis-disease-forum

HEALTHCARE PROVIDERS

Physician Search

Wondering how to find a thyroid doctor? Here are several search engines to find a thyroid expert in your area and find real patient reviews:

American Thyroid Association (ATA)

Search for an endocrinology-thyroid specialist on the American Thyroid Association's online database.

Website: www.thyroid.org/
patient-thyroid-information/
endocrinology-thyroid-doctor

**American Association of Clinical
Endocrinologists (AACE)**

AACE serves as an active voice for
a professional community of clinical
endocrinologists.

Website: www.aace.com

Find an ECNU Endocrinologist:
www.aace.com/resources/
find-an-endocrinologist

**Search For Patient Reviews of
Doctors (MDs)**

A free website allowing patients
to read and submit reviews of
providers.

Website: www.ratemds.com

Web MD

This online publisher of health-related
information, also offers a search for
doctors.

Website: www.doctor.webmd.com

Natural Medicine Providers

Natural medicine practitioners focus
on addressing the underlying cause
of your disease/illness, and typically
incorporate supplements and lifestyle
changes in treatment plans.

**American Academy of Anti-Aging
Physicians (A4M)**

1801 North Military Trail, Suite 200
Boca Raton, FL 33431

A4M promotes anti-aging medicine
as an approach to age related disease,
and educates providers.

Website: www.a4m.com

Phone: 888-997-0112

**American Association of
Naturopathic Physicians (AANP)**

818 18th St. NW, Suite 250
Washington, DC 20006

AANP is a national professional
group whose members are licensed
naturopaths.

Website: www.naturopathic.org

Email: programs@naturopathic.org
(general inquiries)

Phone: 202-237-8150

**The Institute For Functional
Medicine (IFM)**

505 S. 336th Street, Suite 600
Federal Way, WA 98003

IFM is an organization that educates
providers and promotes functional
medicine.

Website: www.ifm.org

Email: info@ifm.org

Phone: 800-228-0622

OTHER HELPFUL WEBSITES

Compounding Pharmacies

Compounding pharmacies prepare
specially prepared medications, which
are designed to meet patients' specific
needs.

**Professional Compounding
Centers of America**

9901 South Wilcrest Drive
Houston, TX 77099

PCCA is an independent, multi-faceted organization whose members are independent pharmacists. The website has a section for patients seeking information, as well as a search tool to find a compounding pharmacy.
Website: http://www.pccarx.com/
Compounder Search Tool: www.pccarx.com/contact-us/find-a-compounder
Email: customerservice@pccarx.com
Phone: 800-331-2498

Prescription Medication

Whether or not you have insurance, you may be able to find particular medications at a lower cost by using the following web and app based service:

GoodRx
A website and app that provides comparison pricing for prescription medications and offers discount coupons.
Website: www.goodrx.com
Phone: 855-268-2822

Environmental Resources

Environmental factors play a role in AITD. These organizations are useful resources for patients who want to learn more about environmental factors and health.

The Environmental Working Group
436 U St NW #100
Washington, DC 2000
EWG is a nonpartisan organization involved in research/advocacy related to human health and the environment.

Website: www.ewg.org
Phone: 202-667-6982

International Academy of Biological Dentistry & Medicine
19122 Camellia Bend Circle
Spring, TX 77379
IABDM is an organization that is comprised of dentists, doctors, and other health professionals who advocate caring for the whole person.
Website: https://iabdm.org
Phone: 281-651-1745

Food and Nutrition

These organizations are sources of information regarding harmful GMOs, chemicals, and how to read and understand food labels.

Center for Food Safety
660 Pennsylvania Ave., SE, #402
Washington, DC 20003
The Center for Food Safety is an environmental advocacy organization that seeks to limit harmful food production techniques and organic and other sustainable forms of agriculture.
Website: www.centerforfoodsafety.org/about-us
Email: office@centerforfoodsafety.org
Phone: 202-547-9359

Food and Drug Administration (FDA)
10903 New Hampshire Ave
Silver Spring, MD 20993-0002
The role of the FDA is to protect public health through supervision of food safety, prescription medications, and other products.

Website: www.fda.gov/food/labelingnutrition/ucm275409.htm

Phone (General): 888-463-6332

Center for Food Safety and Applied Nutrition: 888-723-3366

Vitamin and Supplement Information

There are several websites and consumer reports available that have reliable and independent reviews of different vitamins and supplements.

ConsumerLab

ConsumerLab.com, LLC
333 Mamaroneck Avenue
White Plains, NY 10605

Conducts tests and publishes results for health, wellness, and nutritional products.

Website: www.Consumerlab.com

Email: subscription@consumerlab.com

Phone: 914-722-9149

Consumer Reports

101 Truman Avenue
Yonkers, NY 10703

Paid membership organization that works to provide consumers with truth in the marketplace.

Website: www.consumerreports.org/vitamins-supplements/what-usp-verified-and-other-supplement-seals-mean

Email (online form): www.consumerreports.org/customer-care/email-customer-care

Phone: 800-333-0663

Organic Newsroom

Organization that provides the public with articles regarding positive role of quality organic products on their health and well-being.

Website: www.organicnewsroom.com/best-supplement-brands

Email: info@organicnewsroom.com

About the Authors

Brittany Henderson, MD, ECNU is board-certified in internal medicine and endocrinology, with advanced training in thyroid disorders, including Hashimoto's thyroiditis, Graves' disease, thyroid nodules, and thyroid cancer. Originally from Cleveland, Ohio, she graduated in the top 10 percent of her class at Northeastern Ohio Medical University, where she received the honor of Alpha Omega Alpha (AOA). She completed her endocrinology fellowship training under a National Institutes of Health (NIH) research-training grant at Duke University Medical Center. She then served as Medical Director for the Thyroid and Endocrine Tumor Board at Duke University Medical Center and as Clinical Director for the Thyroid and Endocrine Neoplasia Clinic at Wake Forest University Baptist Medical Center.

She has received multiple prestigious grants from the American Thyroid Association (ATA) and ThyCa (Thyroid Cancer Survivors' Association, Inc.). Her work has been featured on the cover of Thyroid and in many other scientific journals, including *Endocrinology*, *Gut*, and *Oncotarget*. She desires to improve quality of life for those living with thyroid disease both through novel research and medical guidance. For patients living with Hashimoto's disease, she believes that knowledge is power.

Her current clinical practice is located in Charleston, South Carolina, and is dedicated to patients with thyroid disease. She specializes in autoimmune thyroid disease, thyroid nodules, thyroid cancer, ethanol ablation, and advanced minimally invasive techniques. In addition to using a mainstream medical approach, Dr. Henderson also uses complementary medicine to explore underlying root causes of thyroid disease. Visit her website for more practice details: www.drhendersonmd.com.

Dr. Henderson can be found on Twitter and Instagram with the handle @DrHendersonMD, or the hashtag #WYMKAHashimotos. You can also visit her on Facebook at facebook.com/drhendersonmd.

Allison Futterman is a freelance writer who has been published in print and online. She's written human interest, food, travel, profile and writing craft pieces. Her work has appeared in *Philanthropy*, *The Writer*, *Charlotte*, *Winston-Salem Monthly*, and *Today's Charlotte Woman* magazines, among others. Online, her writing can be found on the websites *The Nervous Breakdown*, *Talking Writing*, *Brevity*, and *People of Charlotte*. Additionally, she contributed to the Charlotte Observer for several years. She has a bachelor's degree in communications from Hofstra University and a master's in criminal justice from the University of North Carolina at Charlotte.

Allison is also a patient with chronic medical issues: chronic fatigue syndrome (CFS), fibromyalgia, and Hashimoto's thyroiditis. After years of struggling with illness, she found a true partner in health with Dr. Brittany Henderson. Writing through the lens of their real-life doctor-patient relationship, Allison and Brittany seek to bring that same knowledge to others looking for help and hope.

Allison can be found online at www.allisonfutterman.com.

Index

What You Must Know About Women's Hormones

Your Guide to Natural Hormone Treatments for PMS, Menopause, Osteoporosis, PCOS, and More

Pamela Wartian Smith, MD, MPH

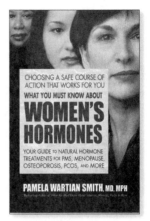

Hormonal imbalances can occur at any age and for a variety of reasons. While most hormone-related problems are associated with menopause, fluctuating hormone levels can cause a variety of other conditions. *What You Must Know About Women's Hormones* is a clear guide to the treatment of hormonal irregularities without the risks associated with standard hormone replacement therapy.

$17.95 US • 256 pages • 6 x 9-inch paperback • ISBN 978-0-7570-0307-3

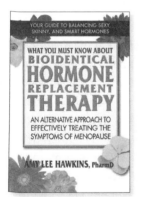

What You Must Know About Bioidentical Hormone Replacement Therapy

An Alternative Approach to Effectively Treating the Symptoms of Menopause

Amy Lee Hawkins, PharmD

Although normal and natural, menopause can cause severe symptoms, ranging from insomnia to depression. Because standard hormone replacement therapy can increase the risk of heart attack, stroke, breast cancer, and blood clots, women often choose to go untreated even when menopausal problems profoundly impact their lives—or they did, until now. Dr. Amy Lee Hawkins offers help through bioidentical hormone replacement therapy (BHRT), which can effectively diminish menopausal symptoms without the dangers of synthetic drugs.

$ 17.95 US • 192 pages • 6 x 9-inch paperback • ISBN 978-0-7570-0380-6

Your Blood Never Lies

How to Read a Blood Test
for a Longer, Healthier Life

James B. LaValle, RPh, CCN

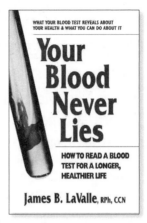

A standard blood test shows how well the kidneys and liver are functioning, the potential for heart disease, and a host of other vital health markers. But most of us cannot decipher these results ourselves or even formulate the right questions to ask—or we couldn't, until now. In simple language, Dr. LaValle explains all of the information found on these forms, making it understandable and accessible so that you can look at the results yourself and know the significance of each marker.

$16.95 US • 368 pages • 6 x 9-inch paperback • ISBN 978-0-7570-0350-9

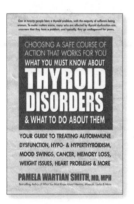

What You Must Know About Thyroid Disorders & What to Do About Them

Pamela Wartian Smith, MD, MPH

It is estimated that one in twenty people have a thyroid problem, and that the majority of sufferers go undiagnosed for years. But it doesn't have to be that way. *What You Must Know About Thyroid Disorders & What to Do About Them* begins by explaining the many functions that the thyroid performs in the body. It then goes on to discuss common thyroid-related disorders and symptoms, including hypothyroidism, hyperthyroidism, excess weight gain, thyroid cancer, and more. Finally, Dr. Smith explains each disorder's cause and common symptoms, diagnostic tests, and both conventional and alternative treatment approaches.

$16.95 US • 224 pages • 6 x 9-inch paperback • ISBN 978-0-7570-0424-7

**For more information about our books,
visit our website at www.squareonepublishers.com**